I hope you enjoy and learn
from my story
Charles Price "Chad"

Can You Feel It in Your Bones?

How a Doctor's Quest Uncovered the Hidden Benefits of Silicon for Bone Health

by Charles T. Price, M.D.

Can You Feel It in Your Bones?
by Charles T. Price, M.D.

First Edition
Cover and interior design by Piotr Zmuda
Editorial assistance by Mike Yorkey
Illustrations by Keri Caffrey

Institute for Better Bone Health
300 N. New York Avenue #2519
Winter Park, FL 32790
1-888-745-4225
www.bonehealthnow.com

ISBN 13: 978-0-9855035-0-5
1. Nutrition. 2. Health.
Printed in the United States of America

To request more copies or make bulk purchases of *Can You Feel It in Your Bones?*
contact the Institute for Better Bone Health.

Important Notice

This book is not intended to provide medical advice or to take the place of medical advice and treatment from your personal physician. Readers are advised to consult their own doctors or other qualified health professionals regarding treatment of their medical problems. Neither the publisher nor the author takes any responsibility for any possible consequences from any treatment, action, or application of medicine, supplement, herb, or preparation to any person reading or following the information in this book. If readers are taking prescription medications, they should consult with their physicians before beginning any nutrition or supplementation program.

Statements related to dietary supplements and foods discussed in this have not been evaluated by the U.S. Food and Drug Administration.

These statements in this book about consumable products or foods have not been evaluated by the Food and Drug Administration and are not intended to diagnose, cure or prevent any disease. The publisher is not responsible for your specific health or allergy needs that may require supervision. The publisher is not responsible for any adverse reactions to the consumption of food or products that have been suggested in this book.

Dedication

To my wife, Pam, who has been my raison d'être since the first time she appeared in a school doorway, and to my mother, Frances Price, who gave me life in more ways than one.

Acknowledgements

There are too many people to thank for *Can You Feel It in Your Bones?* I apologize to anyone who was inadvertently left out.

That said, I would like to specifically thank the following people:

Thanks to my orthopedic colleagues who listened to the science and found it compelling in spite of their initial skepticism.

Thanks to my wife, Pam, who accepted my mental and physical absences, but understood that I was intensely absorbed in a fascinating subject. Pam has always enabled me to pursue my dreams.

Thanks to my children, Travis and Janet, and César Alierta, who became like a brother to me, and to my relatives, who shaped me and helped me become more open-minded.

Thanks to those who read various drafts of this manuscript and provided insightful criticism and suggested improvements: my brother, Alan; my father, Dave; and my colleagues Ken Koval and Josh Langford.

Thanks to those who are named in the book for their contributions as well as graphic designer Piotr Zmuda for his artistic abilities.

Thanks also to Mike Yorkey for his contribution to the written words and to the organization of the book. Mike was a great listener, and his experience as a writer and editor were invaluable.

Finally, thanks especially for the Divine Guidance when it was needed most.

Table of Contents

Part I: The Quest

Why This Book?

Why would a pediatric orthopedic surgeon—whose specialty involves surgery on infants, small children, and adolescents—take an interest in osteoporosis, a condition of weakened and brittle bones in older people? Furthermore, why would he write a book on the benefits of silicon for bone health and also form a company to produce a different bone health product?

The answer starts with a story about my mother, known as "Tutu" by many who loved her.

You would have liked or even *loved* Tutu if you had known her. Her friends thought the world of her, and the hungry-for-affection girls who filled her arms at the House of Hope—a home for troubled teens in Orlando, Florida—

absolutely adored Tutu. She touched thousands of lives during her ninety-three years on Earth.

I loved her as well, but then again, every son loves his mother.

You see, Frances Turner Price was called Tutu by her grandchildren, and the young people who loved her because someone gave her that name and it stuck. The reason it stuck is that "Tutu" means "beloved elder" in the Hawaiian language, and she had that effect on people. Raised the daughter of a Methodist minister, she grew up investing herself in others and loving everyone she came into contact with. She was recognized as "Mother of the Year" for the state of Florida in 1995—at the spry old age of eighty.

Frances was born in Clearwater, Florida, in 1915, into a well-to-do family. Her father, despite the limitations of an eighth-grade education, owned a coffee company that imported flavorful coffee beans from Cuba. Then one day, at the age of thirty-one, Arthur Fred Turner—or "Fred" to his friends—heard God's distinctive call to sell everything and go into the ministry. It was as if Jesus' words to the young rich ruler—"Go, sell all that you own and come follow me"—were directed at him.

Fred Turner heeded that call when Frances was a young girl. Her father sold Triumph Mills—a coffee company that was one of Tampa's most important businesses at the time—and directed the proceeds into the Methodist church. Then he entered the seminary and eventually became the pastor of First United Methodist Church in Orlando, where Pastor Fred "married them and buried them" during a lifetime of ministry to others. He was a frugal soul known for owning just two dark suits—wearing one while the other was at the cleaners.

Besides growing up as a preacher's kid, Frances was greatly impacted by reading *The Magnificent Obsession*, a 1929 novel by Lloyd C. Douglas. The book was based on the true story of a neurosurgeon who performed good deeds secretly, and thereby invoked and bestowed spiritual power. Throughout the rest of her days, giving unconditional love and doing nice things for others would become my mother's "magnificent obsession."

Frances met my father, Charles David Price—who went by Dave—at Florida Southern College in Lakeland as dark war clouds formed over Europe. They fell in love and were married after graduation in 1941, five months before Pearl Harbor thrust the United States into the Second World War.

Dad, raised a Florida farm boy, always wanted to become a doctor but didn't have the money. As soon as the war broke out, the U.S. needed more doctors in addition to fighting men. The Army was offering an accelerated program for battlefield surgeons. Dad enlisted and qualified for the program. He was assigned to the Army Specialized Training Program and attended medical school as a Private First Class.

They moved to New York City, where Dad started his medical studies and Mom worked as a registered dietitian at Columbia University Medical Center. Their first child and my older brother, Alan, came along in 1944, and I arrived fifteen months later as Dad was finishing up his internship at Grady Memorial Hospital in Atlanta, Georgia. I'm told that we lived in a tiny one-bedroom apartment near the hospital, where Dad was on call thirty-six out of every forty-eight hours. That's why he and his colleagues were called interns-in-residence. Pay was $10 a month plus room and board.

By the time Dad was ready for the war zone, World War II was nearly over. He reported for duty in July 1945, following the defeat of Nazi Germany and just weeks before two atomic bombs forced Japan to surrender. Even though the global conflict was finally over, Dad served his time as a surgeon and then worked at a Veterans' Administration Hospital before going into private practice back in Florida.

They bought their first house in 1954, in Winter Park—a small town with brick streets on the outskirts of Orlando that was founded as a destination resort by wealthy New England industrialists at the turn of the 20th century. Our home was a modest concrete block rancher situated among lovely oak and pine trees. We had no air conditioning, but then again few dwellings or public buildings did before the late 1960s.

Our single-story house, painted gray, had double-hung windows that were always kept wide open during the summer months so any lingering breezes could pass through. An attic fan was usually on to keep the hot, sticky air moving. Alan and I drank iced tea, lots of cold water, and cooled off by jumping into a nearby lake. After dark, we'd go frog gigging with our flashlights.

Summer nights could be miserable for sleeping, however. The temperature would sometimes hover in the mid-80s until after midnight, and my brother and I—we shared a bedroom with a double bunk bed—would fall asleep wearing little clothing and no top sheet. The bottom sheet, however, would stick to our sweaty bodies, and pools of moisture formed under our backs and arms. Mosquitoes were sometimes an itchy problem, even though we had screened windows.

Late summertime—when we were back in school—was the worst. The weather was so hot in late August and September that our bony arms would leave a sheen of sweat on our desktops. All that perspiration turned the oily varnish into a tacky mess, which meant you had to be careful where you put your writing and math papers when the teacher gave you an assignment in class.

Mom did two things during high school that greatly impacted me up to this day. The first was when she insisted that Alan and I learn to type during summer school. She issued this directive in the early 1960s, a time when typing was seen as "women's work" and the idea of a "personal computer" was science fiction stuff.

I don't know which was worse—going to summer school in that blasted heat or banging away on those old manual typewriters. Today, I'm thankful she made me take typing because I can knock out eighty words a minute and hit all the punctuation and number keys consistently. I typed all my papers in college and medical school, which probably helped my grades and saved a lot of money back then.

The other thing happened during the spring of my junior year of high school after I attended a presentation given by the American Field Service (AFS). This was a new program for international cultural exchange where students would come from abroad to live in the United States for a school year. The local AFS representative asked if anyone would be interested in hosting an exchange student for the coming school year, saying the experience would "broaden your outlook on the world" and be a lot of fun. It would be challenging because of the additional expenses, but also because of cultural differences with a young student from a foreign land living in your home and sharing your space.

Since Alan was planning to attend Emory University in the fall, his top bunk bed was available, so the idea of having an exchange student sounded adventurous and exotic. Remember, this was in 1962, the heady days of the JFK's "New Frontier" and the Peace Corps. The advent of jet travel during the 1950s made faraway lands much more accessible, but few Americans had visited Europe or had contact with Europeans prior to 1962.

I went home that afternoon, determined to convince my mother that we should apply for the program to have an exchange student live with us for a year. All my arguments were lined up as I put my books on the kitchen counter. While snacking on an apple—Mom, the dietician, was big on healthy snacks— I hesitantly told her about the AFS presentation, and how I thought it would be great if—

"Let's do it," Mom said. Just like that, she agreed to have an exchange student live with us for the school year.

The next day, Mom dropped by school to fill out the necessary paperwork. The AFS matched us with a boy my age from Zaragoza, Spain. His name was César Alierta, and he lived with us for nearly a year. He couldn't even go home for Christmas or Easter break because of the cost and distance. In that sense

César was a real pioneer, leaving everything familiar behind him to travel to a foreign country, live with a foreign family, and speak a foreign language.

I know that César never forgot how my mother loved him during the school year he lived with us. She not only provided affection, trust, and unwavering confidence in him, but she reminded César that life was about following your passion, whatever that might be.

César turned out to be a very good student at Winter Park High. Following high school graduation, he flew back to Spain and served in the military, which he was required to do. Then he graduated from his hometown University of Zaragoza with a law degree and returned to the United States to earn his MBA at Columbia Business School in New York City. Then it was back to Spain, where César started a meteoric climb up the corporate ladder.

He became a financial analyst for a large Spanish bank, Banco Uruijo, and then struck off on his own when he founded Beta Capital, a venture capital company. That led to a position as chairman of Tabacalera, a very large Spanish tobacco company that was established in 1636, making it the oldest tobacco company in the world. Tabacalera was also owned by the Spanish government and had an inefficient management structure. The government wanted to modernize the company and then convert it to a publicly held corporation. César was the right man for that job.

Sure, heading up an iconic Spanish tobacco company that produced popular brands like Ducados Rubio and Fortuna was a huge feather in his cap, but you should have heard my mother give César all kinds of grief through her letters and transoceanic phone calls. She got after him because his company was peddling cigarettes—or "cancer sticks" as Mom used to call them. She wanted him to get out of the tobacco business as fast as he could.

César listened politely, but for him, cigarettes were a commodity, and he had a job to do for Spain. Nonetheless, after three years, he left Tabacalera to become chairman of Telefónica, where he's been the president and CEO since

2006. Mom was thrilled by César's move because Telefónica was not a tobacco company, and she knew he was following his passion as a business leader. Telefónica, headquartered in Spain, is a multinational broadband and telecommunications provider in Europe and Latin America. Operating globally, Telefónica is the third largest telecommunications provider in the world with more employees than the U.S. Navy. We're talking one very *huge* company.

César and I remain close friends to this day, and he told me that much of his business success can be traced back to the year of high school he spent with us. Why does he feel that way? Because he not only understood the Spanish way of doing business, but he could also think like an American, which gave him an additional advantage in the boardroom. When César started to make his mark in the Spanish business world in the 1970s, the direct, American-style business practices stood in contrast to how commerce had always been conducted in Spain, where nepotism was common and the players were more guarded about their business interactions.

But having César in our home taught me something, too—about getting outside your comfort zone and expanding your horizons, lessons that I carried into my adult life and medical career. My exposure to César ingrained in me at a young age that brilliant people and new ideas are universal. In the 1970s and '80s, a time when many physicians in the U.S. looked inward for medical innovation, I was open to traveling to Europe and bringing back new and unfamiliar concepts of caring for and treating patients.

Little did I understand that Mom's quick decision would be a positive influence on the rest of my life and also that of an unknown stranger.

The Long Road to Becoming a Doctor

After César and I graduated with the Class of '63 at Winter Park High School, I followed my brother to Emory University in Atlanta. Going to the same college as my brother was never an issue. Even though we were only fifteen months apart, Alan and I had always gotten along great, even though he was the athletic one and I was the more studious type. There was no sibling rivalry, and I considered him my best friend.

I entered Emory as a pre-med student with a single-minded objective: to become a doctor like my father. Dad didn't push me to become a doctor, but he did push me to become the very best I could be. He is a wonderful father who loves me dearly—Dad is ninety-five years old and still mentally as sharp as a tack—but he still has a perfectionist streak. While I was growing up, he encouraged excellence and celebrated my achievements, but there was always room for improvement. What I mean is that if I came home with a five As and one B on my report card, he'd congratulate me on the As and then ask me why I got the B.

I joined the same fraternity as Alan, and one semester we couldn't find roommates we liked, so we roomed together—just like we did growing up. Some of our fraternity brothers at Alpha Tau Omega razzed us pretty good, but that was one of the easiest semesters either of us ever had. We didn't have any conflicts about studying, sleeping, neatness, or our taste in music. (We were both Beatles fans, but really loved hearing the soul music of Motown—Sam Cooke, Smokey Robinson and the Miracles, and The Temptations—coming from our record player.)

Besides working hard and getting the right grades in courses like organic chemistry and biology, I wrote love letters to my high school sweetheart, Pam Odell, who was attending Duke University. We had met back in 10th grade when she appeared in the doorway of my English class on the first day of school. Her eyes met mine, and attraction bells gonged loudly inside my head. A coy smile covered her face as she glanced my way and slipped into the desk in front of mine. Her hair smelled fantastic. I didn't know her name, but I was whipped right there.

I was so smitten that it took until roll call to realize that her choice of desks had not been the signal I hoped it was. It was only then that I remembered we were sitting in alphabetical order. Her last name began with an "O" and mine with a "P." No matter. She was the one for me. She just didn't know it yet.

I wouldn't say that it was puppy love—a phrase made popular in a song by Paul Anka in 1960—but to use the vernacular of the times, we went "steady" off and on throughout high school and attended Senior Prom together.

Our relationship was tested, however, when it was time to go off to college. While there was never any doubt that I would follow Alan to Emory University because of their great pre-med program, Pam had set her sights on Duke University to study economics. Plus, her mother told her to never marry a doctor because he would be gone all the time.

 That's why it took me a few years to convince Pam that our love-at-first-glance could last a lifetime. After she said yes to my proposal, we married in the summer of 1967—also known as "The Summer of Love," thanks to what was happening in the Haight-Ashbury neighborhood of San Francisco. We exchanged wedding vows two weeks after graduation from college with our undergraduate degrees in hand. Next stop: Baylor College of Medicine in Houston, Texas, where I had been accepted into med school.

All our possessions fit into the back seat of a Ford sedan for the drive to Houston. We planned to become the traditional doctor's family of the late Sixties where the wife worked to put the husband through medical school and then stayed home to raise a family. Things didn't quite turn out that way, however.

We were happy to find a one-bedroom efficiency apartment, but money was so tight that we sold the Ford two-door and bought a Volkswagen Beetle to get better gas mileage. Soon, my young wife realized that her mother had been right: being married to a doctor *did* mean spending a lot of time alone. I didn't have much choice. Medical school in the late Sixties meant forty-four hours of classroom and lab work each week, including four hours on Saturday mornings.

Nights and weekends were consumed with anatomy dissections and studying at home or at the library.

Those of us who wanted to excel—I included myself in that camp—knew we'd better plan an additional forty hours for study each week. I was determined to become an orthopedic surgeon, even though the third- and fourth-year clinical rotations for surgery required me to be at the university hospital at 4:30 a.m. and stay until the following day at 6 p.m. With such a brutal schedule, I was home every other evening, but I was too exhausted to do anything but sleep.

For these and other reasons, young marriages during medical school often fail. Spouses grow resentful because they feel that they are carrying too big a burden for a payoff that's many years in the future. Some couples grow apart as they enter different spheres of life: while the physician gains knowledge, stature, and a career in medicine, the wife pursues short-term employment and the duties of managing the home. Fortunately, my partner-in-life decided that the conventional path was not for her. Pam decided to go to law school and pursue a career of her own.

Remember, this bold move happened before the "women's lib" movement. Prior to the 1970s, women rarely became professionals or had aspirations for an independent career. Those who did choose to become a doctor or a lawyer needed higher scores on entrance exams and greater effort in the classroom to succeed because women were expected to fail—or quit the profession after children came along.

Pam not only excelled in law school at the University of Houston, taking night classes, but she still worked full time to support us. She managed our limited budget, stretching every dollar and putting us through both graduate schools. To bring in a few extra dollars, I worked during vacation times, sold my own blood, and served as a paid experimental subject for research projects at the medical school. That's all I could contribute since my class work and studies gobbled up ninety hours a week.

For several years, we shared an apartment and slept in the same bed, but we only saw each other awake on Saturdays and Sundays—times when we both needed to study. Saturday nights were our only time for relaxation. Since we didn't have enough money to go to a movie, we often got together with friends and played penny-ante poker on Saturday nights. Pam and I got pretty good at Texas Hold 'em, but no one went home with more than a couple of extra dollars.

Going into Private Practice

All the hard work paid off when I graduated seventh in my medical school class (out of sixty-five) at Baylor College of Medicine. Next was one year of internship and four years of orthopedic residency. Pam and I both knew what direction we wanted to go—back to our home state of Florida. Fortunately, the University of Florida in Gainesville had an excellent law school and an excellent orthopedic residency program. During residency training, the sub-specialty of pediatric orthopedic surgery seemed the most fulfilling, but that would require another year of training after orthopedic residency.

Pam wasn't finished, either. She transferred to the University of Florida Law School, but it was a long haul for her. She had to complete nearly two more years of courses at the University of Florida at a time when our first child, Travis, was born. For her bar examination, she was in her eighth month of pregnancy with our second child, Janet. Back then, the proctors had never experienced a near-term pregnant woman in their midst, so they were very nervous about her taking so many bathroom breaks. But it all worked out.

Meanwhile, after an extra year of training in children's orthopedic surgery at the Scottish Rite Hospital in Atlanta, we were able to return to Florida for good when I went into private practice in Orlando.

You'll learn more about my career in pediatric orthopaedic surgery, but upon our return to the Orlando area, Pam made a pact with me. She knew my heart was in academic practice within a university setting—developing new operating techniques, conducting research, and teaching the next generation of doctors. I had been offered a great position as a faculty member at the Scottish Rite Hospital, and I wanted to stay. Private practice, however, paid much more than academic pursuits. There wasn't a medical school in Orlando, but Pam longed to return to the Orlando area to be near family.

Pam suggested that we take the difference in salary between private and academic practice and do some things to help people by creating my own academic practice in Orlando. Her commitment allowed me to hire my own research assistants and publish medical papers. (My first paper published was "The Non-operative Management of Congenital Clubfoot.") The extra money allowed me to present my research at scientific conferences around the world. She helped set up a study and library that was the envy of many orthopedic departments—before the era of the Internet. Her support gave me the opportunity to volunteer on advisory boards, perform community service, act as a visiting professor, and give speeches before community groups.

In many ways, Pam and I were both influenced by the "magnificent obsession" of my mother, who, until her death in 2008, constantly helped others reach their goals. Mom influenced others, too. There was the young man who loved to fly and wanted to become a pilot, but didn't have the means to pay for flight school. Mom enabled him to follow his dream. After a short stint as a commercial pilot for a regional airline, he joined the Navy as a fighter pilot and went on to win the Top Gun competition, followed by a distinguished military career that included flying missions over Iraq. There were others who benefited from Mom's largesse: computer engineers, opera singers, artists, travel agents, and tennis players. She put two young men through seminary, paying for their tuition and books.

Mom's volunteer work at the House of Hope was one of her greatest joys. In the mid-1980s, she met Sara Trollinger, who worked with emotionally handicapped junior high students in the Orlando area and also taught teenagers in the Orange County Juvenile Detention Center. As part of the social service "system," Sara soon learned that the system was a revolving door for those teenagers. They needed a loving, stable family-like environment—like a group residential home—where the teenage residents could learn to accept responsibility, submit to authority, and get along with peers and adults.

Sara talked to five friends about her dream of starting a group home for troubled teens—and one of her early supporters was my mother. They managed to scrape up enough money to buy a well-worn house that became a home to Sara and a half-dozen teenage girls. Miracle after miracle occurred, large and small, like the time when Mom donated a nice conference table that was a perfect match for some chairs that Sara had received from someone else. Finances were so tight the first year that Mom and a couple of other volunteers held garage sales and put on fundraising spaghetti dinners so that Sara could buy groceries and pay the bills.

A big break for the House of Hope came in 1985 when President Reagan flew to Orlando to dedicate the new Epcot Center at Disney World. During the return trip to Washington, D.C., aboard Air Force One, an aide handed the President a copy of the *Orlando Sentinel*, which just so happened to have a feature story about the lives being changed at the new House of Hope. Moved by what Sara Trollinger and volunteers like my mom were doing, President Reagan reached into his briefcase, pulled out his checkbook, and wrote a $1,000 check to the House of Hope from his personal account. Then he penned a nice note to Sara Trollinger and asked an aide to mail it off.

Mom usually devoted one day a week to the House of Hope girls. She'd "adopt" three or four at a time and spend most of the day with them—taking them shopping for clothes, running errands, and just listening to them open up about their lives over burgers and fries at Fuddruckers®.

She asked these girls—many who were living on the streets after their parents abandoned them—questions like, "What is your dream? If you could do anything, what would that be?"

And then she'd try to make that happen for those teen girls. She wanted them to have a chance at this thing called life. This was all part of her "magnificent obsession."

Here's one more story that meant a lot to me. In 1990, President Reagan and the First Lady, Nancy Reagan, agreed to visit the House of Hope, which had grown to nineteen girls at the time. The President, who had finished serving his second term, took a walking tour of the facilities and then participated in a gala fundraising event at a downtown hotel ballroom.

For a $5,000 donation to the House of Hope, you could shake hands with the President and First Lady and have your picture taken with them. Mom splurged and wrote that check, but she insisted that I, along with my high school-aged son, Travis, meet the Reagans and have our picture taken with them. (The limit was two people.) Despite my protestations that she should have *her* picture taken with the President, she wanted my son and me to share that experience. I do know that Travis's brief encounter with President Reagan and First Lady Nancy Reagan made a strong impact on him.

The pictures of Travis and me with the Reagans wound up in frames that Mom kept by her bedside. I still remember the thrill of shaking hands and looking President Reagan in the eye and thanking him for his service to our country. More than twenty years later, Travis remembers that event as one of his treasured memories of Tutu's love.

We had many other cherished memories, of course. But, what happened in the next few years began to open my eyes about the ravages of osteoporosis.

2

Mom's Battle with Osteoporosis

A few years after meeting the President and First Lady, Mom was honored as "Mother of the Year" in Florida. She was proud of the recognition, which I felt was well-deserved. Shortly after receiving the award, however, she shattered her kneecap when she tripped on a step at church. She was eighty years old, and this was the third accident that she had suffered since the Reagans were in Orlando in 1990. The first incident was a compression fracture in her back after being bounced around on an all-terrain four wheeler.

Now, you may be wondering, *What was your seventy-eight-year-old mother doing riding a four-wheeler?* Well, she wasn't driving—her sixteen-year-old grandson, Travis, was in the driver's seat when they hit a hidden dip. You might be thinking they were on a road, but Travis liked to go off-road, exploring in some low-lying wooded areas along a nearby river. Travis had asked Tutu if she wanted to go with him, and being the adventurous type, she said yes.

After she recovered from her ATV injuries, she was rear-ended by a drunken driver while she was stopped at a traffic light. That produced more compression fractures of her spine. Those three or four fractures debilitated her movements rather significantly and probably contributed to falling and breaking her kneecap.

Mom's gait quickly became more stooped. She hunched over when she walked. It didn't take long to notice that she had trouble standing up straight. A first-year student in medical school could make the call from across a crowded ballroom: Mom displayed all the classic signs and symptoms of advancing osteoporosis.

Mom had her own physician, who put her on the latest treatment protocols. As a concerned son and as an experienced orthopedic surgeon, I kept an eye on the situation and encouraged her to walk, take calcium and vitamin D supplements, and do the things that are known to most doctors. Her physician gave her a prescription for bisphosphonates, which is an antiresorptive medicine that slows or stops the process that dissolves bone tissue. Slowing the rate of bone thinning reduces the risk of broken bones. She took her bisphosphonates regularly, but somehow that didn't seem to help her.

In fact, for the last fourteen years of her life, my mother lived an increasingly painful existence as her bones became weaker. On top of doing a number on her kneecap and suffering multiple vertebral compression fractures, she also broke her wrist and ankle in minor accidents.

Pain was her constant companion. Even though she hobbled around and had to sleep in a chair most nights, her spirits never sagged and she rarely complained. At the time, I remember wishing that more could have been done about her bone loss, which was taking its toll on her skeleton. She literally shrank before my eyes. Mom, who had been a tall lady for her era—five feet, ten inches in height and 140 pounds—diminished to five feet, six inches.

Walking became more difficult as she developed a pronounced stooped-over gait. Feeling like *something* needed to be done to help her walk, I found a backpack device from Japan that acted as a counterweight for those hunched over from osteoporosis. I asked Mom to wear the backpack, and she agreed to give it a try. The backpack shifted her center of gravity and straightened her posture—at least somewhat—but she still had a tendency to walk with a pitched-forward gait.

Mom was a trouper and wore the counterweight backpack whenever she had a lot of walking to do, like the times when we took family outings to Disney World or the Epcot Center. She didn't like wearing the backpack in public, however. Also, the device wasn't comfortable, and she felt like her walk was unnatural. As Mom turned ninety and beyond, her health sank even further, but she never held a pity party for herself. Other than her bones, she was a picture of perfect health and mentally sharp.

That was soon about to change.

Mom Takes a Hard Fall

In December 2007, I was serving as chairman of the organizing committee of the International Pediatric Orthopedic Symposium being held in Orlando. This annual conference is sponsored by the American Academy of Orthopedic Surgeons and the Pediatric Orthopedic Society of North America.

This symposium is a premier educational event in the world of pediatric orthopedics, but please don't get the idea that the physicians have time to sun themselves next to the hotel pool or visit Mickey and Minnie with their families. Almost all of the 350 or so pediatric orthopedic surgeons—including the one hundred physicians coming from more than twenty-five countries—

travel alone to Orlando for this intense four-day event that begins at 7:30 each morning and keeps going strong until half past six each evening.

Besides chairing the conference that year, I was also part of the sixty-physician faculty, helping to organize workshops, surgical skills demonstrations, and discussion groups on subjects like spine deformities or congenital hand malformations. As chairman of this conference, I reflected that Pam had been right about returning to Orlando and pursuing our passions from "home."

During a faculty reception on the first evening, I received a phone call from my father, who relayed distressing news from Winter Park Memorial Hospital: Mom had sat down on one end of a small bench at their retirement center—and promptly tipped over sideways. Even though Mom had fallen only two feet, she had broken her hip.

I knew immediately what this news portended. Cold statistics flashed through my mind: three out of four elderly patients never recover completely from a hip fracture, and nearly one in four will die within a year of the fracture because of complications. Despite all the advances in modern medicine, the death rate in the year following a hip fracture had not improved in the past forty years. In other words, my ninety-two-year-old mother was in big trouble.

With great concern, I informed the conference committee that I needed to go to the hospital for a family emergency and they would have to find others to run the conference and fill my speaking slot. With that, I hit the ground running and hopped on the interstate for a quick dash toward Winter Park.

What makes a broken hip such a serious problem among the elderly is not the broken hip itself, but the issues surrounding it. First of all, old bones don't heal very quickly. As much as I'm amazed at how fast the broken bones of children knit together, I'm cognizant—and saddened—by how difficult it is for the fractured bones of seniors to heal.

These types of breaks are known as "fragility fractures" in doctor parlance because they occur from a fall of standing height or less. Trying to fix these fractures in the operating room is like trying to put Humpty Dumpty back together again. The bones can be so thin that screws and plates to repair the damage may not hold the bones together long enough for them to mend. Walking is often delayed because the repair isn't strong enough to support the body's weight.

When active seniors are suddenly bedridden following a fracture and subsequent surgery, they often develop a urinary tract infection because they are too weak to use a bedpan. They are also at risk for delirium, bedsores, and pneumonia. They lose their appetite, which starts the dominoes toppling like toy soldiers lined up in a row: a lack of appetite results in weight loss, which results in a loss in body mass and muscle, which results in overall weakness, which results in feebleness, which leaves the body vulnerable to illnesses and infection.

I was hoping that Mom could beat the odds, just like she did when she was hit with cancer decades earlier. She had developed thyroid cancer in her early thirties after receiving too many bursts of X-rays that she shouldn't have gotten in the first place—500 rads of radiation as treatment for adolescent acne. Radiation treatment for acne wasn't uncommon in the late 1930s when she was a teenage girl, but fifteen or twenty years later, doctors began noticing a big uptick in the number of young people coming down with thyroid cancer.

Some died because the overzealous use of X-rays—before the hazards were fully known—opened the door to cancer. In Mom's case, my dad noticed something early enough to have a chance at a cure. Surgeons removed her thyroid, and then she was put on thyroid medications, which she faithfully took all these years. The cause of her cancer was never a topic of conversation, probably because she survived, but it was always in the back of my mind as a physician. Perhaps that personal knowledge made me a little more aware of possible long-term effects from any medical treatment.

Mom survived thyroid cancer, but falling and breaking her hip was a far different health challenge due to her advanced age. This time around, she didn't heal as well. Her broken hip never fully mended, and she could barely shuffle along with the aid of a walker. Her balance was too precarious to chance walking on her own.

Mom lost considerable strength from the lack of exercise and spent more time in a chair, reading or watching television. Ten months after her fall, she experienced an intestinal obstruction, most likely because of her non-ambulatory existence. Because of Mom's weakened state, her doctors tried to relieve the pressure in her intestinal tract without surgery. For a while, they seemed to be having some success, and Mom did not experience too much discomfort.

I'll never forget the last time I saw her alive. Pam and I were visiting Mom when my adult son, Travis, dropped by. He had been a regular visitor, too. Travis and his grandmother enjoyed each other's company because they shared a good-natured sense of humor.

Travis told her that she needed to get well so they could go out and "paint the town"—which put a smile on her face. "We'll find some hot spot and go dancing," Travis promised.

She looked at him with a knowing smile that seemed to say she had different plans that were fine with her. When we left that evening, she seemed okay.

Several hours later, Mom suffered a massive bowel infarct—which means the bowel suffers the loss of its blood supply, much like a stroke. She lost blood pressure, fell asleep, and never woke up again.

My father Dave, my brother Alan, and I were were at her bedside when she passed into God's glory. We were comforted by the fact that my mother—also known as Tutu, Frannie, and Fran to others—had lived a long, rich life that included sixty-seven years of marriage, raising two boys, enjoying three grandchildren, and impacting thousands of people outside her immediate family.

Mom's memorial service at First United Methodist Church in our hometown of Winter Park was packed with appreciative friends and family members who spoke of the positive impact she had on their lives. For several weeks after her death, I received heartfelt letters and memories from dozens of people who were unknown to us, but whom she had touched in a positive manner through her personal ministry.

In the back of my mind, though, I wondered if she would still be with us if her bones had not become so brittle from osteoporosis. All my years as an orthopedic surgeon had not helped her—not one bit.

That feeling hit home even harder in the next few months because I learned that my wife, Pam, might be headed down the same path. Mom's battle with osteoporosis was over, but another was about to begin for Pam.

3

Silicon Comes into the Picture

One possible answer for Pam's bone health had already appeared, although I didn't recognize the connection immediately. At the time of my mother's fall and broken hip, a major part of my practice was the treatment of a condition called *scoliosis*, or curvature of the spine. Several years earlier, I had been one of the first surgeons in the United States to perform a new method of surgery that had been developed in France, and that had attracted patients from all over Florida and sometimes neighboring states.

Most scoliosis patients are girls, and the condition usually develops just before the adolescent growth spurt. No one knows what causes scoliosis, but it runs in families to some extent. Scoliosis can also affect boys, infants, and small children, but it's more common in adolescent girls. Girls with mild scoliosis don't need any treatment, but some will need braces. Others eventually need surgery to prevent crippling deformity.

Scoliosis surgery involves fusing anywhere from five to fifteen vertebrae of the spine together and holding them in place with metal rods until the bones grow together. Unfortunately, this procedure stiffens the spine, but there's no other way to control severe scoliosis.

Prior to 1984, surgery for scoliosis required a body cast for six months to help the bones heal together. The method had been developed in Texas twenty years previously, but almost one in ten patients needed more surgery because the bones didn't heal. Surgery in adults was even worse.

Then in 1984 a new method was presented by a French surgeon during a meeting I attended. Much to my surprise, this new procedure was not given much attention by the American surgeons. Maybe that was because it seemed unusual or because it was developed outside the United States.

My exposure to César had opened my eyes to advances in Europe, so I was intrigued and sought out the French surgeons, Yves Cotrel and Jean Dubousset. They had developed a method that used a more flexible rod with multiple attachments so that a body cast was not needed after surgery. Three other surgeons from the United States were also interested.

Each of us visited Drs. Cotrel and Dubousset in France and learned the method firsthand. When I felt ready to perform my first case, I invited Professor Dubousset to travel to Orlando to help with the procedure. He graciously agreed, and the case went perfectly. The news media became aware of Professor Dubousset's visit to Orlando, and my patient made national headlines.

Since then, the Cotrel-Dubousset method of segmental fixation has been improved and has replaced the Texas method. My role was to help introduce this new way of thinking that came from France and then to teach other surgeons how to perform the method.

Even though we had a new method that rapidly advanced the treatment of scoliosis, this was still a big operation that required lots of additional bone to make the vertebrae grow together. The additional bone is taken as a bone graft from the patient's pelvis in a way that doesn't weaken the pelvis. Taking the bone graft was part of the procedure, but it increased the time under anesthesia, added to the bleeding, and caused additional pain that made walking more difficult after surgery.

Many surgeons at academic centers, including myself, were searching for alternatives to taking bone from the patient. The alternatives at the time included artificial bone made from calcium and phosphate, or certain types of coral taken from the ocean, processed into small pieces and sterilized. These didn't work very well because the artificial bone didn't have cells or proteins.

This artificial bone was called *osteo-conductive* because it didn't stimulate new bone and only served as a spacer, or conductor, until natural bone could form. Another alternative was dried, sterilized human cadaver bone from donors who had died in accidents, or who had died from causes that weren't contagious. These cadaver bone substitutes and artificial bone grafts were some of my areas of research.

When our new chairman of orthopedic surgery John Connolly, M.D., arrived from the University of Nebraska, he had already done highly regarded research on the injection of concentrated bone marrow into broken bones that had failed to heal after a fracture. Dr. Connolly had shown that injections of bone marrow could restart the healing process by adding cells and proteins that were needed. When he continued this research in Orlando, we teamed up to include bone marrow with artificial bone grafts for scoliosis surgery.

Dr. Connolly and I soon teamed up to prove that an artificial combination of bone marrow and cadaver bone could be created that worked as well as taking large amounts of bone graft from the patient's pelvis.[1] This worked as well as taking large amounts of bone graft from the patient's pelvis.

This artificial combination consisted of dried, sterilized human cadaver bone mixed with a few ounces of concentrated bone marrow taken from the patient's own pelvis.

Bone marrow looks a lot like blood, but it's different because it has different cells and proteins. The fact that bone marrow is liquid means that it could be taken from the pelvis by a technique that used a special needle designed to penetrate bone. In a way, mixing this with specially processed human cadaver bone was tissue engineering for orthopedic surgery. This method was a big improvement over taking bone graft from the patient's pelvis, but it still used human cadaver bone.

It would be better if this could be done with artificial bone made in a laboratory so we would have an unlimited supply. Artificial bone also just seems more acceptable than human bone, even though the cadaver bone is processed and purified. Such an artificial bone didn't exist, although there were new developments coming along on a regular basis.

During this time, I was keeping up with the latest developments in the field of bone graft alternatives and co-authored another scientific study using some commercially prepared products.[2] Perhaps because of my exposure to César, I also kept a lookout for new developments from other countries.

Then in the summer of 2008, about six months after Mom broke her hip, I read about a different type of artificial bone, recently available in Europe, that could be very significant.[3] What I read that summer put me on the path to become prepared for a second battle with osteoporosis in the family, and eventually on the path of starting a nutritional supplement company.

To explain how this happened, I'll have to get a little technical, but the first thing you need to know is that three principles are involved in successful bone grafts. We've already covered some of this, but here are the three principles:

• **Osteo-conduction,** which refers to something that provides a scaffold or spacer so that bone can form. This is the nature of dried, sterilized cadaver bone. It's also the nature of artificial bone made from a type of ceramic material called *calcium phosphate*. The body recognizes the crystalline structure of these materials and uses it as a scaffold to form bone.

• **Osteo-induction,** which refers to proteins, fatty acids, or chemical molecules that trigger stem cells to become bone cells. These proteins and chemical elements can also attract existing bone cells to the damaged area to begin the healing process.

• **Osteo-genesis,** which refers to living stem cells and bone cells that actually create the new bone.

Bone grafts need all three of these elements in order to stimulate natural healing. When bone graft is taken from one place in a person's body and transplanted into the spine or another place in the same person, all of these elements are present because living bone is being moved from one place to another. Taking the bone graft, however, takes something away from one area of the body and uses it in another area. That can cause some additional problems no matter how it's done.

Dr. Connolly and I had found that a combination of cadaver bone and bone marrow supplied all three of those components because the cadaver bone was the scaffold (osteo-conduction), and the bone marrow added the proteins and fatty acids (osteo-induction) along with the bone-forming cells (osteo-genesis).

As I continued to search for something besides cadaver bone, I read about a new type of material that had been developed in the United Kingdom and made its way to Spain and other countries.[4] This new artificial bone was being labeled as **osteo-promotive.**[5] That was a new term meaning it was a material that promoted or enhanced all three of the normal bone processes without adding proteins or cells.

This was different from the other types of artificial bone substitutes. The bone that formed with this artificial bone was *de novo*—fresh or new again. It was more like an electrochemical process instead of a cellular process that was stimulating bone formation. Even when this was put into muscle and not attached to other bone, it could form new bone.[4] This type of artificial bone was doing something that we hadn't seen before.

This new artificial bone graft substitute was made primarily from calcium phosphate, as others substitutes were, but something else had been embedded into the molecular structure of this bone graft substitute—silicon. The studies said that even though silicon accounted for just 1 percent or 2 percent of the bone graft material, the element seemed to enhance the bone-forming properties consistently and measurably.[6] This development intrigued me, as did the pending news that this new form of artificial bone graft substitute was being prepared for use in the United States.

I was also aware of silicon in the medical world because of something called "bioglass"—a glass-ceramic biomaterial made from calcium salts, phosphorous, and silicon.[7] It was known that bioglass could bond with bone and promote bone regeneration, but it had not been used for bone graft material. The more I studied the science of this material, the more it seemed that silicon offered great bone-building potential.

It was at about this point when Pam's battle—and my second clash—began for bone health.

4

The Second Battle

A few months before Mom went to the hospital for the last time, Pam had noticed some pain in her hands. I took a look at her hands and recognized the signs of arthritis that come with age. She made an appointment with a rheumatologist friend of mine who agreed with the diagnosis, but as part of good doctor care, she recommended that Pam take a bone mineral density test.

Pam underwent a DXA scan, a dual emission X-ray absorptiometry test that is commonly used to measure bone mineral density. The results surprised us: she displayed bone mineral density below normal but not quite low enough to be classified as osteoporosis.

In medical terms, Pam was labeled as *osteopenic* because of her T-scores, which are a method of evaluation. If the bone mineral density is said to have a Standard Deviation of -1 to -2.5, then the bones are said to be osteopenic. A score of anything worse than -2.5 is not good and calls for a medical diagnosis of osteoporosis. Pam showed a reading of -1.0 in her femur and -2.2 in her spine, which meant her spinal column was on the cusp of showing a significant loss in bone mass. If she sustained a fracture, her health could deteriorate in a hurry.

Obviously, Pam was losing bone mineral density. Many women accept osteoporosis as a matter-of-fact occurrence that accompanies the passage of time, and that summarized Pam's attitude. Starting between the ages of thirty and thirty-five, women generally lose about 1 percent of their bone mass each year and bone loss accelerates after menopause when estrogen levels decline.[8, 9]

Since Pam had low bone density in spite of taking calcium and vitamin D, her doctor recommended a prescription medication—bisphosphonates—to slow down the rate of bone loss. The risk of long-term side effects immediately came to mind, along with the minimal good it had done for my mother. Fortunately, we could postpone the treatment for a little while because Pam wasn't in the osteoporosis category yet.

I suggested that we put off the bisphosphonates until I could look into her situation a little more. Silicon bone grafts were fresh in my mind, and it was possible that silicon or some other nutrients could help if calcium and vitamin D weren't getting the job done.

Actually, the DXA scan results were somewhat frightening. Pam's ten-year fracture risk was estimated at 12 percent, meaning she had a one-in-eight chance of breaking a hip, wrist, arm, or a bone in her spinal column in the next decade. This could get worse if her bones continued to deteriorate. Pam was still young in comparison to my mother, and she had time to improve if something could be done soon.

After Pam's news, I started studying the medical treatments and especially the one that had been recommended for her. On the medical side of the ledger, the orthodox view is that bone loss generally can't be reversed, so treatment is aimed at *preventing* further bone loss rather than *rebuilding* the lost bone. The conventional management is to exercise and increase consumption of calcium and vitamin D. These are essential parts of any treatment, especially after the age of fifty, whether prescription medicines are used or not.

Expensive new prescription medicines are now available to stop bone loss, but each one comes with side effects—and some are serious. I couldn't shake the thought that Mom's thyroid cancer was caused by X-rays for acne. Whenever there's a new treatment for a disease that's not life-threatening, my first thought is, *What are the long-term effects?* Bisphosphonates, which my mother had taken, carried the risk of dense but brittle bones, unusual fractures, and possible increased risks of cancer. In addition, deterioration of the jaw following bisphosphonates therapy was a concern.

Hormone replacement therapy showed great benefit but also increased the risk of cancer. There were other prescription treatments and injections for osteoporosis, but it was becoming clear that women with post-menopausal osteoporosis who chose these medical treatments were subjecting themselves to some level of risk. These seemed like the best choices for established osteoporosis or for those at high risk for fractures, but maybe not for someone like Pam who was not as severely affected yet. Perhaps there were alternatives that had received less attention.

Just as I was starting to learn more about osteoporosis, Mom's death hit me like a ton of bricks and I realized that my soul mate for more than forty years was heading down the same path unless something different could be found. I wasn't sure what the solution looked like, but as a physician who harbored a lifelong interest in bones, I was going to try to find out.

The Quest Begins

There was a sense of urgency to read and study everything I could on the subject of osteoporosis. This is the *modus operandi* for anyone who wants to unravel a knotty medical question. Throughout my medical career, deep and concentrated study had provided insights that weren't always obvious.

Dr. Richard Feynman, an American physicist and Nobel laureate, described the process of discovery in his book *Perfectly Reasonable Deviations from the Beaten Track.* He said the first ingredient was to have a consuming passion to learn everything you could about a subject. After filling your head with facts on the topic and any related subjects, Dr. Feynman predicted that revelations would come your way at unexpected moments.

I had the passion for this quest, but I needed the facts on this topic and on any related topic. In the realm of osteoporosis that would be impossible. No one could read everything or learn everything about osteoporosis. That meant that there would be gaps in knowledge for even the "experts" who had studied the field for their entire careers. My gaps would probably be larger than theirs, but there was also the possibility that some tidbit of information or something new had not been identified yet.

As an orthopedic surgeon, I had studied osteoporosis and attended educational sessions periodically, but my primary concerns were with pediatric conditions and the latest research on topics like bone healing after spinal fusion, fracture healing, and bone tissue engineering.

Now my attention turned to the osteoporosis front. I knew that osteoporosis research had been undergoing dramatic advances, so I needed to dig deeper into the basic science of osteoporosis and develop my own understanding of this common condition.

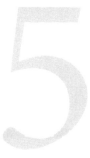

Silicon Gains Ground

The quest began by studying the nearly 500-page report from the U.S. Surgeon General entitled *Bone Health and Osteoporosis*[10]. This was published in 2004 and was the most comprehensive work available on the subject. Richard H. Carmona, M.D. was the U.S. Surgeon General, and he had called together dozens of experts to compile the report. It covered every aspect of osteoporosis and was more complete than any single textbook about osteoporosis. I also purchased two additional textbooks about osteoporosis and read them because repetition is important for learning.[11, 12]

Besides textbooks, I already had a remarkably complete orthopedic library at home, thanks to years of journal subscriptions. Now that trove of research was coming into play as a resource for the study of osteoporosis.

In addition, the Internet placed massive amounts of information at my fingertips. Even obscure publications could be purchased for one-time use from journals intended for veterinarians, biochemical engineers, epidemiologists, and nutritionists. As a professor of Orthopedic Surgery at the University of Central Florida College of Medicine, I could also tap right into our medical school library with access to online textbooks and almost limitless numbers of medical journals in all areas of specialty.

Although I spent most evenings and weekends reading and studying in my home office, I loved every minute of it. I was in my element of learning, learning, and learning about an aspect of bone health that was getting to the molecular level of where the process really began. I found it all fascinating and proved once again that the more you know about a subject, the more it captivates you.

So to recap, during the winter of 2008, I was caring for children on a daily basis, conducting research, and teaching during my day job. Then, I'd come home and learn more about osteoporosis at nights and on weekends. Although orthopedic surgeons deal with the consequences of broken bones, it is the internal medicine doctors who actually prescribe medications and treat the condition, so I had a lot of reading to do. Questions formed in my mind, but one that wouldn't go away was, "How does silicon influence bone formation?"

I sifted through the archives and read original papers, much like a biblical scholar might learn Greek or Hebrew to read the Scriptures in the original language. This approach had been fruitful and revealing in my previous work, and once again this strategy proved invaluable.

After reviewing osteoporosis from almost every angle, it seemed like lesser-known nutrients like silicon might hold a key. Trying to answer that nagging question about silicon proved to be productive immediately.

It's known that bone forms when load is applied to it because small charges of negative electricity develop that attract calcium, in a form called *hydroxyapatite*, to the bone protein.[13-15] This electricity that develops when bone or other types of crystals are put under pressure is called *piezoelectricity*. This was first identified by Japanese researchers and was used by a company called Electro Biology Incorporated (EBI) to create very precise electromagnets that could reproduce the forces that stimulate bone formation.

These tiny electrical forces also explain why jumping, weightlifting, and other forms of exercise can help build bone when healthy stress is applied to the bones. Those activities generate negative piezoelectric forces, but no one knows exactly how.

Then, one evening while reading about silicon, it dawned on me that silicon is widely used in the electronics industry because of its electrical properties. Could silicon enhance or amplify the piezoelectric forces in bone protein? If silicon is concentrated in the bone protein, this could mean that silicon might help attract calcium to bone for mineralization.

Searching deeper into the medical archives, the earliest mention of silicon and bone health appeared in a 1970 article published in *Science* that was authored by Edith M. Carlisle, Ph.D.[16]. In that first publication, Dr. Carlisle reported that she had microscopically sampled various regions of bone in mice and rats. The sampled areas were analyzed for silicon, calcium, and other elements.

Dr. Carlisle reported that the bone-forming sites contained up to *twenty-five* times more silicon than the more mature adjacent sites. She also noted that silicon levels gradually decrease as calcification occurs. Thus, she concluded that silicon is important during the initiation of bone mineralization.

I felt like a person staring into a millstream and finding gleaming bits of shiny gold. This experience was exactly what the Nobel Laureate Richard Feynman had described about revelations coming your way at unexpected moments.

When I read Edith Carlisle's work more than forty years later, the light bulb went on just like Richard Feynman said it would. I didn't know if silicon was a key to osteoporosis, but it had to be a meaningful component for bone health. If silicon helps initiate bone mineralization, this would also explain why silicon-treated artificial bone was showing improved results for surgical procedures.

More reading turned up a couple of dozen recent scientific studies about the beneficial effects of silicon on bone formation, bone repair, and all aspects of bone health, not just in the bone graft substitute arena. I had already asked Pam to hold off on filling her prescription for drugs to treat her looming osteoporosis, but now I asked her to increase her intake of silicon. That wasn't as easy as it sounds, but we'll get to that later.

As part of my study of silicon, I went back to the basics and learned all that I could about this nutrient, which was the eighth most common element on the planet and the second most abundant in the Earth's crust.[17, 18] Pure silicon rarely occurs in nature because it has a strong affinity for other elements. The combined forms of silicon and oxygen are the basic makeup of sand and rocks in the form of silicon dioxide.

Silicon dioxide is also called *silica* and has limited nutritional value, especially in the form of sand because sand can't be digested. Silicon also shouldn't be confused with silicone. Silicone is a synthetic rubber-like compound that is used for medical purposes, sealants, and lubricants. Silicone also can't be digested. Silicone breast implants have been controversial, but in 2011 the FDA approved them again for use in the United States after an exhaustive safety review.[19]

Silicon, however, doesn't seem to have any toxicity.[20-22] The United States National Institutes of Health and the European Food and Drug Safety Commission have not found that any amount of silicon causes adverse effects.[21, 22] Even when large amounts have been fed to animals, including pregnant animals, no harmful effects have been identified.[18, 21] The body needs silicon like it needs water, and the body is also capable of getting rid of excess silicon under normal circumstances.[23-25]

Silicon is not only abundant in nature, but it has special electrical properties that are useful for computer chips and circuit boards. This explains why the U.S. high-tech industry—Apple, Google, eBay®, and Cisco Systems, Inc.—located between San Francisco and San Jose is known as "Silicon Valley."

After becoming aware of this element in the bone graft literature, it seemed like my forays into other aspects of bone health kept turning up more and more about silicon and its role in reversing bone loss. My search yielded a bonanza of scientific evidence that silicon was essential for bone formation.

A comment by one author, however, captured the rest of what I was uncovering when researcher Ronald G. Munger wrote, "The preoccupation to date with calcium has resulted in less emphasis on the role of other nutrients in bone quality and osteoporosis."[26] That pretty much summed up what I was finding, too. Other nutrients besides calcium and vitamin D were very important for bone health, but those were not being widely promoted in medical circles. Silicon seemed to be the most overlooked, so I focused on that first.

Some of the current scientific literature about silicon was easy pickings—like research on animals and several convincing population studies showing that higher levels of dietary silicon intake were associated with increased bone mineral density.[27-38] Orthopedic surgeons or internists aren't expected to read this type of research until it has some practical applications for specific treatments with known doses and methods of delivery. It seemed like there was a lot of evidence, but no one had connected the dots.

Dr. Carlisle had continued her research with several additional studies that established silicon as an essential factor necessary for bone formation. Her last paper appeared in 1981 when she gave more proof that silicon improves the quality of bone matrix, or the scaffolding on which bone is calcified, and that silicon makes the matrix more receptive to calcium so it can become hard bone.[39] Somehow, silicon was attracting the calcium to the bone matrix and helping the bone mineralize.

Over the next twenty years, silicon research was spotty. The only major study on silicon and bone health appeared in 1993 when Hott, et al. evaluated the effects of silicon supplementation on post-menopausal osteoporosis in lab animals.[27] These researchers reported that silicon, when added to the diet, caused increased bone formation and decreased bone resorption. The silicon was actually increasing bone density, and that was a very interesting observation.

Somewhat surprisingly, nothing much happened on the research front for seven more years until around 2000, when the benefits of silicon for bone health started cropping up from various and differing sources that clearly identified silicon as an essential and important element for bone health.

For instance, one population study from Massachusetts showed that the intake of more than 40 mg of silicon per day was associated with increased bone density, yet the average dietary intake for postmenopausal women was 18 mg per day.[22, 36, 40] I also learned that in certain areas of China and India, where the diet was rich in grains harvested from silicon-rich soil, the general population received an average intake of 150-200 mg of silicon a day.[41, 42]

Could this mean that there were fewer hip fractures in China and India, the two most populous countries on Earth?

That was an intriguing question. I looked for the published data on the worldwide frequency of hip fractures. Sure enough, those areas of China and India *did* have the lowest frequency of hip fractures—and by a wide margin compared to Western civilizations.[43]

Silicon supplementation had also been studied in post-menopausal women. One study was conducted twenty years ago using intramuscular injections of a soluble form of silicon.[44] Treatment was compared to other medicines including bisphosphonates. At the end of four months, the silicon group had improved femoral bone density that was even more than the bisphosphonates group.

Another study using dietary silicon followed by bone biopsy showed improved bone volume.[45] Studies that used smaller doses of silicon compounds, or shorter periods of time, have been inconclusive, although one study showed that the femoral bone density was maintained in the silicon group, but not in the placebo group.[46, 47]

Further study led to the fact that converting hard water to soft water—which is prevalent in the United States—removed natural silicon by a process called *flocculation*.[48, 49] Learning about this was more evidence that we are likely to be silicon deficient, at least in comparison to other cultures.

Next, I turned to veterinary science and agricultural science in pursuit of every possible lead. It's known that feeding supplemental silicon to chickens and quails improves the strength of eggshells.[50, 51] Extra silicon also strengthens the bones of quails so they don't break during mechanical processing.[52] Silicon added to farm-raised trout produces larger fish with healthier bone structures.[30]

Everywhere I looked, silicon showed beneficial effects for bone health. One study in race horses was particularly meaningful since my daughter, Janet, has been around horses since she was a little girl and is a professional riding instructor today. She not only instructs kids on the basics of how to properly ride a horse, but she also teaches youngsters the elements of discipline, preparation, sportsmanship, and mastering a talent.

When horses get a broken bone, it's life-threatening—like a hip fracture in an older woman. Thoroughbred race horses are especially prone to broken legs, and famous ones have gone to their graves on the racetrack. I still remember the time when the filly Eight Belles finished second in a field with nineteen colts at the 2008 Kentucky Derby, but moments after crossing the finish line, she suddenly collapsed on the race track. Her two front ankles were broken. A tarp was raised to shield the proud race horse from onlookers and TV cameras, and then Eight Belles was euthanized by injection.

This study in race horses used the highest level of scientific research called a randomized, prospective, controlled blind trial.[31] This means that different diets were given to different groups of race horses. In this experiment, there were four groups with different levels of dietary silicon. They were fed and studied for a year and a half with careful documentation of training schedules, race times for similar distances, injuries, and actual race results.

What made this study even more valid was that no one knew which horses received the silicon supplements in their food until the end of the study when the different groups were identified. For eighteen months, the food supplements were delivered in packages marked with just the group number so that each horse received the right diet for that group. The packages were prepared at the University of Kentucky veterinary school, and the ingredients were kept secret from everyone managing the horses.

When the horses were two years old, the code was revealed and the information was compared. The horses that received the silicon supplementation had stronger bones, faster track times, fewer injuries, and more training distance without lameness.

What struck me reading reports like this and reports in medical journals was that the medical community was not yet aware that silicon could be important for bone health. I turned back to the U.S. Surgeon General's *Bone Health and Osteoporosis Report*, which called attention to the increasing problem as the Baby Boomers reach retirement age.

U.S. Surgeon General Richard Carmona declared that those entering middle age were not only at great risk of developing bone diseases like osteoporosis, but also of experiencing *fractures* from declining bone health. In other words, unexpected slips and falls could result in greater numbers of cracked elbows, broken ankles, and hip fractures—even for those ten or fifteen years younger than Pam and me.

While the Surgeon General was warning of the dangers of osteoporosis for those middle aged and older, he also called attention to the fact that 85 percent of adolescent girls and 65 percent of boys do not get enough bone-building nutrients, such as calcium and vitamin D, to support normal bone health. I viewed this statement as a wake-up call to parents because the peak bone-building years happen during childhood and adolescence. A twenty-year-old who has 10 percent more bone density than average postpones the onset of osteoporosis by more than a decade.

While there was a lot to like in the Surgeon General's assessment, I couldn't help but notice that silicon was not presented or discussed anywhere in the document.[10] This comprehensive report, prepared by a panel of experts, identified twenty nutrients that had effects on bone health, but silicon was not one of the twenty nutrients that were discussed.

Was I missing something, or were all these experts missing something? Of course, I doubted myself totally and thought about forgetting the whole thing—like someone who imagined seeing Bigfoot or the Loch Ness Monster.

Then it dawned on me that the report, released in 2004, had probably been compiled in 2003 or even beginning in 2002. I was reading that report in 2009, meaning that most of the rising flood of research about silicon began *after* the Surgeon General's report was issued. The bulk of silicon information that I had found was so recent that it couldn't have been included in this important document.

It was like silicon was hidden in plain sight.

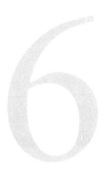

Connecting the Dots

While contemplating this information about silicon, a thought arrived in my consciousness: *Someone needs to connect the basic science to clinical application, and that hasn't been done for silicon.*

That someone, I realized, could be me—a realization that hit me in the chest like a medicine ball. While I knew that eventually science would triumph with or without me, I was also aware that it might take years before the benefits of silicon and lesser-known nutrients would find their way into everyday management of osteoporosis.

My career plan was to stop doing surgery when I turned sixty-five, to slow down a bit for travel, golf, and more time with grandchildren. Giving up surgery would also give me time to teach orthopedics at the Med School and manage a program created by our children's hospital for prevention of a common hip problem in babies. This program is called the International Hip Dysplasia Institute and was generously funded by the nationally known comedian, Larry the Cable Guy.

You read right—Larry the Cable Guy. That's another story in itself, but hip dysplasia is the most common abnormality in newborn infants, and "Larry" had challenged us to form an international group of experts to see what we could do to change that.

Now I could hear a voice in my heart calling me to do one more thing before I "retired." This new, invigorating, and personal quest to prevent osteoporosis had been placed on my doorstep like an abandoned baby.

Spreading the word about silicon and nutrition for bone health seemed like a perfect fit for my talents as a senior orthopedic surgeon. Orthopedic surgery really does require stamina, excellent eye-hand coordination, and fine motor skills that decline with age. Eyesight is perhaps one of the most unappreciated qualities of a good surgeon. Until the age of forty-five, my eyesight had been 20/10. I could spot different species of birds on the wing, including almost any variety of duck, just by their pattern of flight, size, and general appearance.

The gift of 20/10 eyesight was an advantage in surgery, but it is possible to compensate with eyeglasses, optical lenses called "loupes," or operating microscopes. High-quality reading glasses were all I needed in surgery for the past fifteen years. Nonetheless, there can be a culture of silence about an older surgeon who has lost his or her skills and continues to operate.

There are a few excellent surgeons who continue to operate after the age of sixty-five, but many continue too long. Their colleagues are reluctant to tell them they've lost their edge. I planned to "hang it up" before someone told me that I should.

Quite frankly, I could have packed things up, purchased a condo on the beach, and read interesting books the rest of my life while getting plenty of vitamin D from the sunshine, but something was telling me that I should look at my "easing into retirement" years in a whole different light—as a grand opportunity to contribute more through my skills, experience, and availability.

I also heard Mom's voice deep within me, saying, "To whom much is given, much is expected." Thus, I willingly put aside thoughts of slowing down and welcomed the opportunity to move forward and help those suffering from poor bone health and diseases like osteoporosis. This would become my "magnificent obsession."

The way I viewed things, here was a chance to accomplish a few more things that could benefit others.

This quest for a new direction in osteoporosis was cognitive and would fit with my plans to step out of the operating room—except that I needed more time now and not three or four years down the road. I didn't really want to give up my lifelong interest in bones, and this quest could occupy the final phase of my career long after the age of sixty-five. Besides, studying about osteoporosis and basic bone metabolism was fulfilling and personal.

Pam and I had talked about retirement in a few years, but she knew that I'd be bored unless there was something besides golf and fishing to keep me busy. I joked with her that I'd retire as soon as we cured hip dysplasia and osteoporosis. That sounded ridiculous because those two conditions had been recognized by Hippocrates, and there had been little progress towards prevention since then.

In spite of that, it did seem oddly possible that I'd been given the opportunity to introduce some new approaches that might just work.

Pam and I were about to find out.

Coming Up with a Plan

Pam knew how much I'd loved surgery, but she also knew that surgical skills don't last forever. Pam may also have sensed a certain amount of enthusiasm with a new way to approach an old problem.

The typical surgeon's day begins at 7 a.m. in the pre-operative area so the actual surgery can begin promptly at 7:30 a.m. After several cases or afternoon office hours, the surgeon completes his or her paperwork, makes some phone calls, returns to the hospital for post-op rounds, and leaves for home around 7 p.m. or later.

Taking emergency calls is part and parcel of orthopedic surgery, so that requires more time in the hospital. Thus, some surgeons set aside Wednesday afternoons for recreation time. That "afternoon off" is sometimes ridiculed in movies and television shows, but it's well deserved and much needed.

Academic institutions are required to report work hours for faculty as well as residents. The residents are restricted to no more than eighty hours of work in a week, but there are no restrictions on the faculty. My time sheets would show that a typical work week averaged about seventy hours for over thirty years. Stopping surgery would be a big adjustment for me in many ways, but that would give me the time I needed to pursue this new quest.

After talking with Pam on this major career decision, I asked the hospital and my colleagues to make arrangements so I could stop doing surgery. Fortunately, this was a natural transition in our academic program. There's a lot of non-operative care in the field of pediatric orthopedics, so it would actually help the department if someone with my seniority spent more time in clinic and less in surgery. I could still continue my teaching and my service to professional organizations. It would be a fitting conclusion to my career, even though I still had all my surgical skills.

It took several months to wind down my busy practice. My schedule shifted to a normal forty-hour week, and I had more time and energy at night and on weekends to devote to the study of bone health. I was excited by the possibility that silicon and other nutrients might have an important place in the prevention of osteoporosis. If true, that information could help Pam and also help others facing the threat of osteoporosis so they might live better and richer lives in their golden years.

Besides reading the latest clinical research, there was also some useful information in non-medical journals or available on the Internet. Unfortunately, there's also a lot of misinformation on the World Wide Web. Several years previously, I had edited a book for the American Academy of Orthopedic Surgeons that included a chapter on complementary and alternative medicine for arthritis.[53] We included that chapter because medical doctors are interested in nutritional and holistic approaches to medical care. Medical doctors, however, also want to see the evidence for claims of what works and what doesn't so they can give their patients reliable advice.

Doctors are interested in meaningful alternatives to traditional health care. They know that medicinal plants have given us potent medicines including heart medicines, anesthetic drugs, and a cure for malaria, to name just a few examples. Other more recent examples include using aspirin and omega-3 supplements as healthy habits.

Doctors also know that the mind is a powerful source of health or illness, and they understand that the placebo effect can make medicines appear very powerful when meditation, prayer, or relaxation might work just as well and would be safer.

Sometimes doctors may appear to be disinterested in alternative health, but that is rarely the case. What doctors are looking for is a reliable and trusted source of information about complementary and alternative medicine. That is no different from the general public, but the amount of information can be overwhelming. My role would be to try to sort out the truth from the fiction.

As it turned out, there was plenty of solid science showing that silicon has measurable bone-strengthening properties. My reading also uncovered good clinical research about some lesser-known nutrients that are essential for bone health.

I began to include some of this information in lectures about bone healing and in presentations about artificial bone graft substitutes. These were presented during visiting professorships and as an invited speaker at national and international conferences. Each time, the response was very positive and the doctors were hungry to learn more, which lifted my hopes that the role of silicon in bone health was truly useful information.

My long career in academic orthopedic surgery had established some connections with leading investigators for many aspects of bone health.

During this quest, I talked with an M.D./Ph.D. colleague who was doing laboratory research on bisphosphonates and a similar colleague who had reported on cellular functions during bone formation, in addition to publishing a chapter in a science textbook entitled *Bone Injury, Regeneration, and Repair*. Both of these highly regarded physicians were intrigued and told me that they had not considered silicon, but they did agree that silicon was worth a closer look.

My goal was to raise awareness of silicon as an important component of bone health and to stir the pot among those who were in a position to spread the word. A written outline was presented to two other friends who were contributors to the Surgeon General's report on osteoporosis. Both agreed to include silicon in their discussions of bone health. All of this was very encouraging.

Meanwhile, I continued my research. With each passing month, it became more and more obvious that silicon and other nutrients had not received enough attention for bone health.

Most adults in North America need some calcium supplementation but probably not much more than 500 mg a day of extra calcium, as long as it's being absorbed efficiently.[26, 54-56] It becomes an exercise of diminishing returns because excess calcium is poorly absorbed.[10, 57, 58] Also, after menopause, the ability to absorb calcium decreases even more for women.[10, 59] The good news is that other nutrients like boron and vitamin D can improve calcium absorption and reduce calcium loss.[60-62]

In addition, other nutrients could affect the absorption, utilization, and retention of calcium in the body. As Dr. Munger noted, a balanced approach to nutrition was probably more important than forcing large doses of calcium in hopes of overcoming osteoporosis.[26]

Magnesium is increasingly recognized as an important contributor to bone health. About half of the body's magnesium is in bone, and magnesium is especially important for spinal bone strength.[54, 63-67] Even more surprising is that more than half the people in the United States have inadequate dietary intake of magnesium.[22, 68]

My reading uncovered several reports recommending modest supplementation with magnesium to support bone health.[54, 65, 69, 70] The average intake for women in the United States is 240 mg.,[22] but the National Institutes of Health recommended daily intake of 320 mg for women and 420 mg for men. [63]

An estimation of diet in prehistoric hunter/gatherer societies suggests that daily intake of magnesium was about 600 mg/day for our ancestors.[65, 71] Magnesium is also used in antacids and laxatives, so too much magnesium can lead to diarrhea or abdominal cramping. Modest supplementation with magnesium is safe, partly because excess is either not absorbed or is removed by the kidneys as long as the person does not have kidney failure. One study of women with osteoporosis showed improved bone density when they were given a supplement of 250 mg of magnesium each day for two years.[69]. The message that magnesium is important for bone health is gaining attention, but there's a long way to go for the general public and for doctors to recognize this essential nutrient.

As I kept on learning and studying, a whole new world was coming into view for the first time. I was discovering some strong science in support of silicon and several other lesser-known nutrients for bone health, and my background in research helped me uncover more kernels of truth. Here are a few more that deserve attention.

Boron is increasingly recognized as an element that has several health benefits including bone health.[60, 72, 73] The name *boron* sounds like a metal, but it's not. In fact, boron is a lightweight element that has properties similar to silicon. Boron is considered non-toxic except in very large amounts because it dissolves in water and the kidneys can get rid of excess boron.[22,

74] Boric acid is so mild that dilute solutions are used for eye wash and for minor cuts as an antiseptic.

The precise mechanism of action of boron for bone health is unknown, but boron stabilizes vitamin D and estrogen so they act over a longer period of time.[22, 61, 74] That should be helpful because vitamin D and estrogen are beneficial for bone health. Supplementation with 3 mg of boron per day for post-menopausal women has been shown to prevent loss of calcium *and* magnesium.[73] Increased bone strength has also been demonstrated in pigs fed a diet supplemented with boron.[75] Prunes are a rich source of boron, with approximately 3-4 mg of boron for every three-ounce serving of prunes.[76, 77] A study of postmenopausal women reported that a three-ounce serving of prunes daily for a period of one year improved bone mineral density, but dried apples did not.[78]

Another nutrient, vitamin K, has also been studied for bone health.[79-81] Research about hip fracture risk showed that women who consumed more than 109 micrograms of vitamin K per day had a decreased risk of hip fractures compared to women with lower levels of vitamin K intake.[80] Vitamin K has several different forms, but vitamin K_1 and K_2 are the naturally occurring forms.

Vitamin K_1 is important for coagulation of blood, while vitamin K_2 is more important for bone health.[79, 82] Vitamin K interferes with warfarin, a blood thinner that goes by the brand name Coumadin®, so people taking that type of blood thinner should avoid vitamin K supplements. Otherwise, naturally occurring vitamin K is non-toxic even when consumed in large amounts.[22] High levels of intake do not increase blood clotting, even though vitamin K is important for coagulation.[22]

In Japan, the use of vitamin K for osteoporosis is showing some impressive results.[82, 83] In one study, megadoses of vitamin K_2 more than two thousand times the recommended daily amount were used to treat women with advanced osteoporosis[82]. In that study, the frequency of spine fractures was reduced almost as much as women treated with bisphosphonates. One surprising finding was that the bone mineral density stayed about the same.[82, 84] This suggests that vitamin K_2 improves the flexibility of bones and makes bones stronger without increasing the calcium content.

I was learning that silicon seems to help mineralize the bones, while boron helps stabilize hormones and vitamin K improves the flexibility of bones to make them more resilient and less likely to break.

Other nutrients also play an important role in bone health, and I kept learning more and more about how these nutrients work together in the body. For example, certain proteins improve absorption of calcium from the intestines into the bloodstream.[85] Some of these are found in milk and dairy products. [57, 86] This shows that there are factors besides the total amount of calcium that affect how much calcium gets into your bones.

On top of that, other nutrients influence the amount of calcium that's absorbed, so the incorrect balance of nutrients may prevent some of them from getting into your system.[85, 87, 88] When large amounts of silicon are consumed at the same time as calcium, they can't both be absorbed very well.[35, 87] There's only so much the gut can absorb at any one time as everything passes through. If all the nutrients come through at one time, then the nutrients aren't always digested evenly. This is especially true with calcium and silicon because they compete for the same pathway to get into the body.

What was more worrisome was that some of the nutrients for bone health can be overdone. These include zinc, copper, manganese, and vitamin A, to name just four. A little supplementation is okay, but too much of those nutrients can be bad for your health.

It is widely known that vitamin A supplements can cause birth defects if taken during pregnancy.[22] Also, too much vitamin A can make osteoporosis worse.[22] Just taking twice the recommended daily amount of vitamin A has been shown to increase the risk of hip fracture and decrease bone mineral density.[89, 90]

Copper and manganese are increasingly questioned as dietary supplements.[91, 92] A little is needed for bone formation and for general health, but too much can build up, and some studies suggest that too much may contribute to Alzheimer's or Parkinson's diseases.

Zinc is also important for nerve function, but too much is toxic. An imbalance of zinc in the brain—with too much in some parts of the brain or too little in other parts—is also found in diseases like Parkinson's and Alzheimer's.[93, 94] The right amount of these elements is important, but too much can be unhealthy. The food safety commissions of various countries have recommended upper levels of intake of these nutrients to avoid these and other effects.

Looking at a New Approach

The more I learned, the more it became evident that the right balance of all these nutrients is important. There are interactions that rely on the proper balance of many different systems (including the brain and spirit) working together. As everyone knows, too much of a good thing is not a good thing. Life balance is more important than over-emphasizing one good element.

Unfortunately, not everyone can achieve the right life balance, including myself. Most of us need some help in one or more areas. For bone health, that would be the role of supplements in the form of pills for those of us who don't have a completely healthy lifestyle.

The medicinal chemists, nutritionists, and Ph.D.s have created a wealth of outstanding information, but there is an aspect of being a physician that helps you see how the whole body functions as a living organism.

What happens in real life is that people who are deficient in silicon are likely to be deficient in other nutrients like vitamin D, magnesium, vitamin K, or boron. Studies of large populations may look at dietary intake of silicon and show that those who consume more than 40 mg of silicon have better bone density. What may also be happening is that people who consume more than 40 mg of silicon may also be getting adequate amounts of other nutrients. Likewise, people who consume less than 40 mg of silicon may consume lesser amounts of other nutrients.

That simple observation is why a balanced approach is what's needed instead of searching for the "magic bullet." Once again, I could feel Mom's influence. As I mentioned earlier, she was a registered dietitian, so searching the nutritional literature did not seem as strange to me as it might have to other physicians. In fact, she had been the head dietitian at the Eye Institute of Columbia University Medical Center in New York City.

During the child-raising years with Alan and me, Mom kept her hand in the medical arena when she became the Chief Dietitian at our community hospital where my father was a surgeon. My surgeon father and dietitian mother often debated the merits of certain diabetic diets, post-surgical diet plans, and other aspects of medical care between bites of Mom's casseroles and vegetables. Counting calories and paying close attention to nutritional values were standard dinnertime discussions while I was growing up.

It took a lot of time and effort to identify the most important nutrients for bone health because there is conflicting information. Checking and cross-checking is fundamental to the process of investigation.

After identifying the important nutrients for bone health, the next step was to determine how much of each of these nutrients might help Pam. The recommended daily amounts for general health are reported by the Institute of Medicine of the U.S. National Academy of Sciences.

It seems simple enough to look up the recommended amounts and then see how much to take each day. However, other countries don't always agree with the American recommendations. The European Food Safety Commission makes recommendations for Europe, and there are highly qualified agencies in other countries that make their recommendations. As you might expect, there are differences of opinion about the best amounts for general health. I was interested in that too, but mainly I was interested in the amount needed to reduce the risk of osteoporosis for my wife, Pam.

The recommended amounts fell into a range that made sense for general health, but sometimes that range could vary depending on age, sex, or even by the country making the recommendation. For example, the recommended amount of vitamin D in different countries varied by twice the amount recommended in the United States, and up to five times the U.S. amount was recommended in some reports.[95-98]

So, it was a long process to review as much information as possible from around the world to determine my own recommendations that might help Pam. I certainly didn't want to take any chances with her health, so I tried to determine how much of each nutrient would be good for bone health and compared that to what was already in an average American diet. Also, I wanted my recommendations to be based on needs for women with weakening bones, rather than the generally healthy adult population.

After deciding which nutrients and how much of each might benefit bone health, I started looking for a nutritional product that had those amounts in it. What I found was somewhat surprising to me. It seemed like most of the available products had some of the ingredients that affect bone health, but none had the combination that seemed best to me.

In fact, many had more than the recommended amount—whether more was needed or not. For some nutrients, like vitamin C, vitamin D, and vitamin K, a little more is okay, but for nutrients like zinc, copper, and manganese, or Vitamin A, some had too much in my opinion.

Take zinc, for example. I wondered how much was in the typical

American diet already, and I questioned whether we even need a supplement for zinc. Some papers published in 1979 and 1984 suggested that many Americans were deficient in zinc, but that was based on old recommendations and different dietary habits.[99, 100] Currently, the recommended daily intake of zinc in the U.S. is 8 mg for women and 11 mg for men. It turns out that the average dietary intake in the U.S. is 9 mg for women and 14 mg for men.[101, 102]

So, that means that the typical American gets plenty of zinc in their diet. That's because zinc is found in a wide variety of foods including red meat, lamb, shellfish, seeds, nuts, dairy products, poultry, and beans, just to name a few.

Vegetarians and older people may have insufficient zinc intake, but even after the age of sixty at least two-thirds of Americans have adequate zinc in their diet. Perhaps an elderly person with poor eating habits needs some zinc supplementation, but most do not. Studies in Europe and the United States have shown that more than 90 percent of the population has adequate zinc intake without needing supplements.[103, 104] One study even showed that 96 percent of older people in Europe had adequate zinc intake.[105]

In addition, some studies suggest that more zinc, than 25 mg/day may be harmful.[106, 107] There is some concern that high levels of zinc, intake may increase the risk of anemia and copper deficiency. When I looked at the labels of some multivitamins, many contained 10-15 mg of zinc while one had 30 mg. If that's added to the average dietary intake, a person could exceed the upper level recommended by the National Institutes of Health of 40 mg/day.[101]

I followed the same process for all the other nutrients that I had identified—first deciding how much was good for bone health, then checking to see if that was provided by a typical and average American diet, and then deciding how much was needed to make up the difference.

It turned out that the recommended amount of copper is 0.9 mg/day, and more than half of Americans are already getting 1.1 mg/day in the average diet.[22, 102] The recommended amount of manganese is about 2 mg, and the average American is already getting about 2.8 mg.[22] This means that most Americans are getting enough copper and manganese for bone health and for general health. In spite of that, many multivitamins have extra copper and manganese, and some supplements have several milligrams of each.

The trend toward excessive or unnecessary supplementation may help explain why, in 2011, a report showed increased mortality with some dietary supplements.[108] Zinc, iron, and copper were three of the ones associated with increased mortality rate. Calcium supplements seemed to lower the risk of death.

Pam eats a typical American diet, so I decided to leave zinc, copper, and manganese off the list of supplements for her bone health. They do benefit bone health, but she didn't need extra, and extra might be harmful over the long haul. That seemed especially true for the newest rage in bone supplements—strontium.

Strontium

Strontium needs a special place in this book because reading about strontium raised my eyebrows and shows why medical doctors are sometimes skeptical of the nutritional supplement business.

Strontium immediately caused me concern because it's a metal and is closely related to calcium.[109] Calcium is also a metal. In fact, strontium, calcium, and magnesium are all called "alkaline earth metals" because they have similar properties.

That may sound good, but calcium is important for nerve transmission, muscle function, and other body functions besides strengthening bone. Inviting strontium to come into the body and do those jobs might be an invitation for trouble.

The human body is set up to use calcium and magnesium in specific places and for specific purposes. If strontium is like calcium and magnesium, that similarity might fool the body and allow strontium to take the place of calcium and magnesium. Thus, it might be a bad idea to substitute something for calcium when calcium is the body's first choice.

In Europe, a specific form of strontium called *strontium ranelate* had been patented and used as a prescription medicine for over five years, but the United States Food and Drug Administration (FDA) had not approved it for use in the U.S.

Not everything that comes from Europe is good, and their drug approval processes are sometimes less rigid than the ones in the United States. While the FDA is sometimes criticized for being too regulatory, it did keep thalidomide out of the United States and that saved thousands of babies from terrible malformations of their arms and legs back in the 1950s. All you have to do is Google images of thalidomide babies, and you'll become a big supporter of the FDA. In the case of strontium ranelate, the FDA had not approved it for safe use in the United States. That was enough for me to dig a little deeper.

A scientific study published in the prestigious *New England Journal of Medicine* in 2004 reported that strontium ranelate had demonstrated increased bone density and lower fracture rates for women who took two grams a day for three years.[110] There is other evidence that strontium does create bone and reduce the rate of fractures in women diagnosed with advanced osteoporosis.[111-113] But my first concern is that two grams is a lot of anything that's not normal for the body. Said another way, that's 2,000 mg a day for three years—huge doses in my opinion. My questions were: *Where does it go?* and *What happens to it?*

I also wondered why the FDA had not approved strontium ranelate for use in the United States as a prescription drug to treat osteoporosis, even though it had been used for years in Europe. The full reasons aren't clear, but what I learned gave me enough concern to hope that the FDA continues to be cautious.

First of all, there are no truly long-term studies, and that reminded me of my mother's experience with thyroid cancer caused by radiation to treat acne twenty years before the cancer developed.

As I began to dig through the scientific literature about strontium, the first thing I found was that strontium is not an essential nutrient. This means we can live healthy lives without any strontium[109]. Sometimes very tiny amounts of certain trace minerals are essential and are needed for us to survive. But we don't ever need any strontium . . . nada, zilch, none.

Perhaps this is why strontium is not under homeostatic control.[109] This means that the body lacks the ability to regulate excess amounts of strontium. In the case of calcium for example, the body can regulate the amount of calcium in the blood by allowing the intestines to absorb more or having the kidneys get rid of more, depending on whether there's an excess or not.

The body has feedback loops for regulation of calcium balance. In osteoporosis, those feedback loops may not be acting properly, but at least they exist and can be used for treatment. The body doesn't have any way to regulate the uptake or elimination of strontium, however. That's probably because it's not an essential nutrient, so it acts more like a foreign substance.

A second concern was that strontium can push calcium aside in the nerve endings and substitute for calcium where nerve signals are transmitted.[114] When that happens, the nerve signals are slower because strontium is not the same as calcium.[115, 116] In another study, young pigs were fed strontium and some developed coordination problems and paralysis.[117]

One study of strontium ranelate showed that slightly more women taking strontium complained of memory loss compared to the group taking a placebo.[111] Also, there may be a small but statistically significant increase in the number of potentially dangerous blood clots in the group taking strontium ranelate.[111, 118]

A third concern was that strontium makes the bone X-rays appear denser than they really are because strontium is a heavier metal than calcium.[119] Lead poisoning also makes bones look denser because lead is taken up in bones. Strontium absorbs the X-rays and makes the bones look denser to the X-ray machines and to the DXA scan.

There are ways to adjust the reading of the DXA scan to show the true bone density, but these adjustments are not fully developed, so the DXA scan results may look better than they really are for people taking strontium.[119] Anyone taking strontium in their nutritional supplement should inform their doctor so the reading of the DXA scan can be adjusted; otherwise, it might show a false increase in density.

This ability of strontium to block X-rays is why it was used in early television screens.[120] The early television tubes gave off X-rays, so strontium was mixed into the glass to absorb the X-rays and block the viewers from harmful effects.

A fourth concern came from studies of regions of the world that have high amounts of strontium in the soil and therefore in the diet. Some of those areas have high rates of rickets.[121] That suggests that the strontium can block the normal function of calcium in the bones when taken over long periods of time.[109] Strontium might make the bones denser and more resistant to breaking, but reports show that too much strontium causes deformities and poor growth in children.

A fifth concern was that once strontium gets into the bones, it stays there for years and years and years. One study estimated that ten years after taking strontium, most of it would still be in the bones.[119]

Normally, the entire body has about 300 mg of strontium because it gets into our bodies from the environment.[122, 123] That amount doesn't seem to be harmful, but taking two grams a day of strontium ranelate will increase the amount of strontium in the body to about 30 grams or one thousand times the normal amount.[119] If there are long-term effects of strontium, it will not be possible to reverse the damage after that much is in the bones.

This concern about long-term effects of strontium may be one reason why the FDA has not allowed strontium ranelate to be used in the United States. Since the results of strontium ranelate are similar to bisphosphonates for osteoporosis, bisphosphonates might be a better choice if the osteoporosis is bad enough to need prescription medications.

There was no doubt in my mind that Pam wasn't going to take any strontium in the near future. More and more nutritional supplement companies were rushing to put some strontium in their bone health products, and a few of the promoters were making claims based on unproven assumptions about doses and composition.

When patients bring this type of information to a doctor's office, the doctor often hasn't had time to study the subject to render a good opinion. It's easier to just recommend calcium and vitamin D because those are known to be safe and effective. Maybe ten years from now, strontium will be proven safe and effective, but maybe it won't. I didn't want to risk that for Pam.

What I found on the store shelves for bone health were a lot of products that had too much of these questionable nutrients, especially for someone taking a multivitamin for health benefits besides bone strength. After figuring out the most important elements for bone health, it was time to figure out how much of each nutrient was needed for her fairly typical American eating habits. I wanted something for Pam's bone health that would supplement her diet and supplement her multivitamin without providing too much of anything and without any of the questionable nutrients.

Eating healthy organic foods is the best way to get these nutrients, but few Americans follow the dietary guidelines recommended by the U.S. Department of Agriculture (USDA). The ideal diet would be low fat, low salt, and low calorie and would include five daily servings of fruits and vegetables plus whole grain cereals and breads, milk products, nuts, and a variety of protein sources. That seems unlikely for most of us, even though we'd be healthier if we ate like that.

Insufficiencies in the Average American Diet

Some nutrients needed for bone health are poorly supplied by the typical American diet. Calcium and vitamin D are well-known examples that are often insufficient in today's diets. Some supplementation with those two nutrients is important for bone health, especially in postmenopausal women. Other nutrients that are usually low include vitamin K, boron, silicon and magnesium.

Pam needed some calcium supplementation because most women aren't getting enough calcium in their diet, and she seemed no different. The National Institutes of Health recommends 1200 mg per day for women older than 50 years, but the majority of women in the United States consume less than half that amount on a daily basis.[58, 102] Some multivitamins have calcium but seldom enough to make up the 600 mg difference. Pam needed a little more calcium than her multivitamin but not so much that it might increase her risk of heart attack and kidney stones. I settled on an amount that would meet her needs without going overboard.

What's probably more important than calcium is vitamin D.[62, 85] Not only does vitamin D improve calcium metabolism, it also improves muscle function and that could be important for prevention of falls.[124-126] The recommended daily allowance for vitamin D is 800 IU, but some reports have recommended more.[95, 96, 127] This includes a recommendation from the

Endocrine Society that 1500-2000 IU per day may be needed.[96]

The average American diet provides only 150-300 IU of vitamin D. More vitamin D can be manufactured in the skin with exposure to sunshine, but sunscreen is needed to reduce the risk of skin cancer—and that blocks the formation of vitamin D. Also, we spend more time indoors for entertainment and work than we did fifty years ago. This means that most Americans should be receiving some supplemental vitamin D for general health in addition to the benefits for bone health. Even the American Academy of Pediatrics recommends that vitamin D supplementation should begin for all children by two months of age and continue through adulthood.[128]

In spite of all the evidence that calcium and vitamin D are important for bone health, there is still some controversy whether these two nutrients alone can reduce the risk of fractures. A few studies have shown poor correlation with vitamin D levels and osteoporosis, while others have shown the opposite.[129, 130]

Some reports have found decreased hip fracture rates in women taking supplemental vitamin D, while others have been inconclusive. These conflicting findings may be related to the amount of supplementation. A statistical analysis of multiple research studies was published in the *Journal of the American Medical Association* in 2005. That analysis concluded that higher doses of daily vitamin D supplements in the range of 700-800 IU decreased the risk of fractures, but lower doses of 400 IU were ineffective.[131] This finding along with the recommendation of the Endocrine Society made sense to me, so Pam needed a good dose of vitamin D, but not an excessive dose.

After studying all of this information, I was even more in agreement with Dr. Munger's statement that other nutrients besides vitamin D and calcium were needed in a supplement.[26] Vitamin D and calcium are insufficient in most American diets, so Pam needed more calcium and vitamin D for sure, but some of the other important nutrients were also insufficient in her diet.

According to the Food and Nutrition Board of the Institute of Medicine, more than half the women in the United States have below the recommended level of intake for vitamin K.[22] Since vitamin K is important for bone health and there's no harm with high intake, dietary supplementation with vitamin K seems reasonable for optimum health. In addition, the combination of vitamin K and vitamin D has been shown to improve bone mineral density better than either of those supplements alone.[83]

Another insufficient nutrient is boron. Approximately half the population of the United States consumes less than 1 mg of boron per day.[22] The National Institutes of Health have not recommended a daily amount of boron, but a diet low in boron decreases the effectiveness of estrogen that's important to bone health.[73, 74]

Also, supplementation with more than 3 mg/day has shown improved calcium metabolism, as has increased intake of prunes.[73, 74, 78] Since no toxicity has been reported with increased boron intake, and because most women consume less than 3 mg per day, it would be reasonable to supplement Pam's diet with some additional boron. It was also possible to increase boron intake by eating more prunes, raisins, dried apricots, almonds, or avocados on a daily basis. Pam's eating habits, however, were more like the typical American, so she needed some extra boron.

The recommended amount of magnesium for women over the age of thirty is 320 mg, but more than half of the women in the United States get less than 210 mg per day.[63, 102] That's more than a 100 mg deficit for most American women. Older women may get even less because of poor dietary intake and poor intestinal absorption. It made sense to add some extra magnesium. The need for extra magnesium has been recognized by the medical community for several years, although this need is less widely known than the need for extra calcium and vitamin D.

When you look at it this way, what jumps out at you is that more than half the people in the U.S. are getting insufficient amounts of six major nutrients important for bone health. They are vitamin D, calcium, magnesium, silicon, vitamin K, and boron. On the other hand, most people take in plenty of vitamin C, copper, zinc, and manganese. A small amount of extra vitamin C was added for Pam because extra vitamin C has been shown to improve bone density and decrease the risk of hip fractures in women with osteoporosis.[132-134]

Armed with that information, I took the next step in Pam's nutritional program. I checked her multivitamin, and it had too much of some things and none of the others. Also, calcium competes with silicon for absorption into the bloodstream, so those would likely be more effective if they were taken a few hours apart.[35, 87]

Sound confusing? Well, join the club! It was also confusing to Pam, who has an economics degree from Duke and was second in her class in law school. Plus, it has to be confusing to doctors who don't have time to go through this type of analysis.

Next, I turned my attention to a couple of other nutrients that have been associated with improved bone mineralization, and these are often insufficient in the typical American diet. They were:

• **Inositol**, a carbohydrate that helps slow down bone loss. Inositol occurs naturally in phytates that are in husks of nuts and grains. Too much phytate can interfere with calcium absorption, but some phytate is needed to improve bone mineral density and slow down bone loss.[135-137] The inositol component of phytate seems to be the active part that hardens the bones and make them more resistant to loss.[138-140]

• **L-arginine**, an amino acid that's a chemical building block of protein. L-arginine has a special effect on improvement of microscopic blood circulation and plays a beneficial role in wound healing, fracture healing, hormone secretion, and cellular function.[141-144] Studies where L-arginine, inositol, and silicon were taken together demonstrated increased bone mineral density and increased bone strength.[29, 30, 52]

Eventually, I settled on a group of nutrients, including silicon, but excluded other ingredients like strontium after reading and studying more than 400 scientific papers, several books about osteoporosis, recommendations from several other countries, and the Surgeon General's report. I also reviewed a textbook on orthopedic basic science, talked with some star researchers, combed the Internet, put my findings into lectures for peer criticism, and did a lot of deductive reasoning.

That formed my plan for Pam. Now it was time to implement the plan.

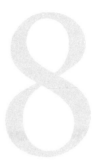

Winning the Battle

During this research period, I had Pam increase her intake of silicon and other supplements. She was already taking vitamin D and calcium before she was told that her bone density was poor, and she needed to keep taking those, of course.

Her exercise was sporadic, however. Sometimes she'd work out for a few weeks on a regular basis, but she still had a busy law practice, so there were often days when there were not enough hours in a day to squeeze in a workout.

The main reason I wanted her to get on some type of weight-training program was because I knew how important it was to prevent the first fracture. The first broken bone for someone in their senior years sends a strong signal that the bones are weak. Indeed, an older woman who has a hip fracture loses bone mass in the *opposite* hip five times faster after the initial injury.[145]

It's also a lot tougher to prevent a second fracture following a first fracture, so it was important to build up Pam's bones so she wouldn't break a wrist, an arm, or a hip. Looking back, it seemed clear that Mom's first spine fracture started a downward spiral of bone loss caused by poor posture, poor balance, weaker muscles, and decreased activity. Pam needed to avoid the first fracture.

I must confess, however, that Pam took the news of her bone density fairly lightly. When she came home from her doctor and told me she had been diagnosed as osteopenic, she commented, "A lot of women my age have low bone density."

Pam was like a lot of women who felt, *Okay, my bones are getting thinner. I'm not too worried about it. I can still drive my car and go to work. I can still play golf. Sure, I'm a little shorter and lost some strength, but what's the big deal? That's what happens when you age. If there's a pill I can take, I'll take it. At this stage in life, I don't really want to change my lifestyle.*

I knew better, which is why I hid my anxiety. I could see the difference in Pam's weakening skeleton in something as simple as hitting a golf ball. She had lost a lot of yardage in the last few years.

Pam was a *good* golfer who had played to an 11 handicap in spite of full-time work as recently as her mid-fifties. She had started playing when she was a little girl and had one of those gorgeous swings that reminded golfers of Patty Sheehan, the two-time U.S. Open winner who fashioned a Hall of Fame career.

On occasions when Pam hit balls at the practice tee, other golfers would drop by and casually ask if she played professionally. She'd laugh it off and then go back to striping 230-yard drives, farther than some men who play regularly. Sometimes she'd really connect and the ball would sail even farther. Remember, this was back in the days before the souped-up Titleist Pro V1 balls and carbon-fiber drivers, so she could really hit the ball pretty well.

Whenever Pam and I traveled on vacation, we'd take our clubs and chase the little white ball around the golf course. As a twosome, we'd inevitably be paired with two other golfers for the round, and I always enjoyed seeing the faces of a couple of guys who walked up to the first tee box only to see that they would be playing with a . . . woman.

The disappointment was written all over their faces. *Today's our unlucky day, dude. We're playing with a woman who can't hit the ball. It's going to be the slowest round ever!*

I'm a high handicapper, just a social golfer, so I'd hit from the white or blue tees with the guys and then get in my cart with Pam and drive up to the women's tee. I could see our playing partners thinking, *Come on, let's get this over with. She'll probably top the ball fifty yards.*

Pam would step onto the tee box, waggle her driver a few times, groove that beautiful swing of hers, and blast the ball down the middle of the fairway with the jaw-dropping crack that only a well-struck ball can make. With the advantage of playing from the ladies' tees, she blew past the guys handily. I would immediately notice a change in our playing partners' demeanor. *Bubba, we're going to have to step up our game here.*

Pam had lost a tremendous amount of distance in recent years. Those towering drives that arched 230 yards before landing softly in the middle of the fairway? She was now lucky to hit it 180—still a reasonable distance for someone her age, but nothing like the days when she brought her "A" game to the course.

Pam was no longer five feet, four inches either. She had shrunk an inch, and some of this was probably related to osteoporosis. To help her turn around her bone loss, I was convinced that she needed to take some type of nutritional supplement that had silicon in it, plus the other nutrients besides vitamin D and calcium.

Finding such a supplement would prove a lot more difficult than I expected.

The Dietary Sources of Silicon

I dropped by our local supermarket and checked out the shelves in the pharmacy section, looking for words like *silicon* or *silicate* on the labels of some of the leading multivitamins.

I really didn't find much. A couple of different multivitamins contained 2 mg of silicon. I read the fine print and saw that the silicon in these multivitamins was silicon dioxide! Silicon dioxide is like sand or quartz, which means that it's not very likely to get into the bloodstream. A chemist could flame the vitamin and prove that there's silicon in it, but what good would that do for someone's bones if the silicon dioxide went right though the intestines and came out the other end without being digested?

Even if the 2 mg were absorbed, Pam needed at least 40 mg of silicon a day—the amount that I believed was the sweet spot. I was fixated on that level of silicon because clinical studies from Massachusetts and Scotland reported increased bone density in the high-silicon group when the daily intake was more than 40 mg a day.[36, 37]

The average American diet provided around 20 mg a day, but most women Pam's age were getting less than that.[22, 36, 40] She had been raised on meat and potatoes and wasn't likely to change her eating habits now, so I needed to find something closer to 30 mg for her every day.

Most of the high dietary silicon levels in the Massachusetts study were achieved through drinking a lot of . . . beer.[36, 48] That's right, beer. Beer is made from barley, and the distilling process captures the silicon from the whole grain.[146, 147] Even non-alcoholic beer is good for your bones,[148-

150] but Pam wasn't a beer drinker. Stocking the fridge with brewskies and asking her to drink a long neck with breakfast, lunch, and dinner just wasn't going to work.

But there were some other reports about dietary sources of silicon. Foods with good amounts of silicon were green beans, spinach, whole wheat, oatmeal, brown and wild rice, and other whole grains,[146] but Pam wasn't eating a lot of those foods in her typical American diet. A fruit with silicon that she *did* like—bananas—turned out to not really help her. The research said that the silicon in bananas wasn't readily absorbed, meaning that bananas weren't helping her bones.[48]

As I continued my search for foods or drinks with strong levels of silicon, I learned that orthosilicic acid is a highly absorbable form of silicon and is in some mineral waters from artesian wells around the world. [150, 151] A study of 207 brands of Italian mineral water reported that 23 percent had more than 10 mg of silicon per liter (approximately a quart), and those with the highest amount of silicon came from volcanic regions of the Italy.[151] After checking around, I found a few brands of mineral water from France that had as much as 30 mg of silicon per liter.[49] Some mineral waters from Fiji had 60 to 85 mg of silicon per liter.[23, 47]

If Pam would drink a glass of silicon-rich mineral water daily—around a pint—I had a strong feeling that we would get the silicon train out of the station. Eating foods with whole grains like breakfast cereals, breads, rice, and pasta would give her some silicon as well.

Pam agreed to eat things like oatmeal for breakfast and consume more whole grain bread. But as we discussed the idea of having her take some nutritional supplements to "cover our bases," I explained that I hadn't found much on the shelf with an effective combination of silicon, vitamin K, or boron, so we were going to have to improvise.

Necessity being the mother of invention, I jerry-rigged a bone-building nutritional supplement program for my wife. Since she was already taking some calcium and vitamin D, omega-3s, and a multivitamin, I added the following nutritional supplements, plus the mineral water:

- 1 capsule of additional magnesium
- 1 capsule of vitamin K
- 1 capsule of boron
- 1 capsule of inositol, even though the recommended daily use on the bottle said three capsules a day (I didn't think that much was needed for Pam.)
- 1 capsule of L-arginine

The calcium, magnesium, and vitamin D needed to be taken at different times of the day than the other ingredients. The L-arginine came in capsules with vitamin B6 and some other things, but that was okay.

I got Pam started with these supplements, but continued my search for something that combined all of these nutrients without going overboard on nutrients like zinc, copper, manganese, and vitamin A.

Still, I couldn't find a nutritional supplement with an adequate amount of silicon in a useful form that would be absorbed. Also, my goal was to find a balanced supplementation protocol rather than taking megadoses of any one nutrient.

Pam was fine with my advice to drink at least a large glass of mineral water daily, although it was expensive and heavy to bring home from the grocery store. Speaking of cost, the expense of purchasing all of the other supplements was fairly high when you added them all up.

There was another issue that raised its head. With this grab bag of nutritional supplements, Pam had more than a half-dozen plastic bottles of vitamins and minerals grouped together next to the sink. Pam drank the mineral water fairly regularly, but she didn't always take the other supplements like she was supposed to. There were a lot of different ones to take, and some of them were supposed to be taken at different times, so Pam had trouble staying with the program.

So what happened after she started drinking her special water, doing some occasional exercise, and taking the other supplements?

A lot.

One year after she began her regimen, when Pam had another DXA scan, the results were impressive. Her ten-year fracture risk dropped from 12 percent to 6.9 percent—a 42 percent decrease. Her bone mineral density actually improved instead of just staying the same or getting worse, which is considered a huge success in the medical world.

Most of the improvement was in the weakest area of her right hip, where the bone is supposed to be thickest, but where she had the most bone loss. That part showed a 50 percent improvement in the T-score. This amount of change without prescription medications was a remarkable achievement and beyond what anyone could expect from going on an exercise jag and taking calcium and vitamin D alone.

As it turns out, silicon was more important for cortical bone of the hips than for the spongy bone that makes up the vertebrae.[34, 44] For the vertebrae, magnesium and other nutrients may be more important than silicon, but something had definitely helped her bone density—and everything pointed to silicon. That improvement gave Pam renewed interest in taking the other supplements, but that was still a challenge because sometimes she was just too busy to sort through all those pills every day.

When Pam's doctor learned these results, though, she was astounded. "What in the world are you taking?" she asked.

"Well, Chad said I should take these nutritional supplements with silicon and a few other things," she answered.

"So you weren't taking any bisphosphonates?" her doctor continued. A year earlier, she had given Pam a prescription for the osteoporosis-fighting medication.

My wife shook her head. The answer was *no*.

When Pam came home and told me about the amazing turnaround in her osteoporosis condition, I knew we were on to something. When you stop and think about it, she actually experienced an increase in bone mineral density although she—like nearly every women past the age of thirty-five or so—could be expected to *lose* bone mineral density year-to-year.

Could this work for others?

That's when the next door opened and reinforced my belief that things happen for a reason.

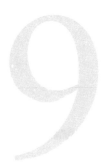

The Third Battle

Just as Pam was finding out that her bone density had improved, the third episode in this battle for bone health began to take shape. My brother Alan asked for some medical advice about his wife, Sue, my sister-in-law. They live just a couple of miles from us in Winter Park.

Sue had been a highly regarded first-grade teacher and once had been named Teacher of the Year locally because of an innovative, award-winning science teaching, program that she had developed. She retired once from teaching but missed the kids so much that she returned to the classroom. When she retired a second time, she became a much-in-demand substitute.

Sue had gone through some health challenges in recent years. A few years earlier, she had broken her ankle and then had two "total knees"—or artificial knee replacements.

One evening, Alan called me and said that Sue was having some trouble with osteoporosis. A few years earlier, Sue had a bone mineral density test to use as a baseline, and when she was tested recently, the report noted that she had experienced a significant loss in bone mineral density over an eighteen-month period. She had lost 17 percent of her bone density in just a year and a half. Her doctor was recommending that she take bisphosphonates, which is what prompted Alan's call to me. He wasn't sure if she should go on them, and he wanted to bounce that idea off me.

Alan's a dentist, so he was well aware of a condition called *osteonecrosis of the jaw* (ONJ) that was cropping up in people taking oral bisphosphonates. If a tooth has to be extracted from a patient on bisphosphonates, the risk of a severe infection is a lot greater than someone who's never taken bisphosphonates. Osteonecrosis of the jaw is a serious malady.

After listening as Alan explained what Sue was going through, I asked him to send me her DXA scan. Reviewing that made it was obvious that Sue's bones were worse than Pam's. Sue showed T-scores of -.8 for the spine and -2.3 for her left hip. (Remember, a score of -2.5 is true osteoporosis, so Sue was perilously close.) Her 17 percent loss of her bone density the last eighteen months meant that her bones were losing calcium at an alarming rate.

What made this all the more worrisome was that Sue had been doing everything she was supposed to do. She exercised at a gym regularly and had done so for the previous four years. She was also taking a multivitamin with extra calcium and vitamin D.

What's more, I knew Sue ate healthy because she and Alan had a vegetable garden and grew most of their own vegetables, herbs, and fruits. Sue was the most health-conscious person I knew. She baked bread and included whole grains and nuts in her daily diet. My brother, Alan, is an avid hunter and fisherman, so they also ate a lot of fish and wild game, including plenty of low-fat venison.

Pam and I love being invited to their home because Sue's meals always include seasonal, home-grown, fresh-picked fruits and vegetables. Thus, I knew Sue was getting plenty of the nutrients like vitamin K and boron. When I asked Alan to tell me more about the foods she ate, it seemed clear to me that the main element missing was silicon.

At this point, I told my older brother what I had been doing for the last year or so—researching silicon and tailoring a regimen for Pam to follow. We had just received Pam's first DXA scan results, which showed a dramatic improvement in bone mineral density.

I recommended that Sue continue taking her multivitamin along with some calcium and vitamin D, but I told Alan that she needed to add silicon—by drinking some silicon-loaded mineral water—to everything else that she was doing. I also encouraged her to eat more prunes to increase her boron consumption.

In this way, Sue was the perfect subject to see what silicon could do. Even though this was only one test case, it was my assumption that silicon was the main ingredient she was missing, and this missing nutrient might be the reason her bones were getting thinner in spite of everything she was doing to prevent that from happening.

When Alan relayed the plan, Sue turned out to be an eager beaver, faithfully drinking her special water and telling everyone else to buy some too. She found the lowest prices by buying in bulk and probably purchased enough liters of water to start her own distribution company. I also had to convince her that she didn't need to drown herself in water. Although I wished Pam had taken her program more seriously, Sue's condition was more threatening.

In September 2011, we learned that Sue was rewarded for her efforts. The absolute bone mineral content in her problematic left hip had increased a whopping 26 percent. That was a marvelous change and way beyond what seemed possible, especially since her bone density had been decreasing in spite of exercise, calcium, and vitamin D. Sue's left hip now had a T-score of -1.0 instead of -2.3.

Her spine density hadn't improved as much as her hip, but there was a 6 percent improvement in her spine. Perhaps she actually needed the additional supplements, so she's now adding some to her regimen, but the silicon seemed to make a big difference for her hip.

The amount of improvement we had seen in Sue and also in Pam meant that silicon combined with other nutrients could have tremendous benefits for bone health. These two experiences exceeded my expectations but matched my hopes.

Every doctor knows that two cases don't prove anything, but the changes in Pam and Sue were dramatic enough to convince me that silicon and other nutrients like boron, vitamin K, inositol, and L-arginine deserved a closer look. Maybe the story of Pam's and Sue's successes could be used to open some doors and hopefully get some osteoporosis specialists fired up about silicon and the lesser-known nutrients.

At least we had two people who were bucking the trend, so that was a good place to start.

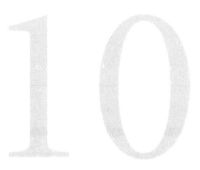

Seeking an Open Avenue

Changing the landscape of osteoporosis now seemed possible, but physicians treating osteoporosis needed to be informed of the whole view of nutrition besides calcium and vitamin D. It also seemed worthwhile to try to convince a pharmaceutical company to create a specific product, based on my research, because the specific product that Pam needed wasn't currently available.

I also wanted something that others could take for bone support, even if they were like Sue with healthy eating habits, or while taking a multivitamin with some of the commonly available ingredients. That could be a difficult task. Pharmaceutical companies have saved millions of lives with their innovations, but each product takes years to develop and requires millions of dollars to prove safety and efficacy before it can be released to the public.

In addition, the wide open field of nutritional supplements was both good and bad. One good aspect is that the safety of vitamins, minerals, and other natural supplements can be determined from existing studies. Another blessing of nutritional supplements is that new findings, like the recent research about silicon, can be applied immediately.

A problem with nutritional supplements is that some supplements are poorly designed or may have harmful formulations. New rules adopted by the FDA are attempting to limit the new and unknown ingredients until they are proven safe.

Another problem is that useful nutritional supplements are difficult to patent for protection of the seller. For this reason, pharmaceutical companies can't put millions of dollars into research and expect to get their money back since other companies might use the research to make a similar product that they could sell at a lower price. This means that there's not much money spent to study new supplements to see if they have the potential to help people.

In spite of these obstacles, it still seemed worthwhile to talk with a drug company about the possibility of developing something different from other nutritional supplements—something that could be added to a healthy diet or to multivitamins for anyone who was already health conscious.

There was plenty of need for such a product. For starters, osteoporosis is responsible for a lot of carnage in this country, and with Baby Boomers like myself leading a huge cohort into the post-retirement years, the problem was only going to get bigger. The statistics show that osteoporosis leads to 1.5 million fractures per year, mostly in the hip, spine, and wrist, according to the U.S. Surgeon General's report.[10]

The condition afflicts more than 44 million Americans—68 percent of them older women who see bone loss accelerate after menopause. One really worrisome statistic is that a woman over the age of fifty has the same chance of dying from a broken hip as she does from dying of breast cancer.[152, 153]

Even when modern medicine gets someone on her feet and out of the hospital after a hip fracture, there can still be more trouble in the coming year. All too often, that first serious fracture can lead to more broken bones, weakness, loss of mobility, and—for the elderly—a downward spiral that can lead to an untimely death.[153, 154]

Surely, there was a health-related company that would recognize the key role that lesser-known nutrients like silicon, arginine, inositol, vitamins K and C, boron, and magnesium play in bone health. These nutrients needed to be put together in a way that would supplement what most of us were getting in our normal diets. In addition, the metals and vitamin A that might accumulate in the body needed to be left out.

After searching the local health food stores, nutrition centers, and the Internet, I couldn't find an appropriate supplement that had what I wanted. If there were a package with these bone health nutrients in the amounts I was looking for, it might help people besides my family members.

You see, I had a formulation all worked up, ready to go. All it would take was a company that would make the product, and we would probably have a nutritional supplement that could really make a difference. I was even willing to hand over the formulation to a dietary supplement company if they caught the vision of what needed to be done.

But as I found out over the next year, none would catch the vision.

11

Exploring the Possibilities

I didn't have a strong idea about how to go about finding a company that could be convinced to make a new nutritional product, but I know what Mom would have said—"Follow your passion, son." There were other influences, too, from growing up on the outskirts of Orlando, in Winter Park, during the 1950s and '60s. These influences told me that anything is possible.

Back then, the United States and the Soviet Union were locked in the "Space Race," and the nation's attention during that time was focused on a spit of sand known as Cape Canaveral located just fifty miles east of Winter Park. Cape Canaveral was chosen because the land stuck out on the side of Florida, and the surrounding area had very few people living around there. In the early days of launching rockets, there was a real fear that a rocket could explode or fall back to Earth—which they did with alarming regularity during my childhood.

Oranges, cattle, and rockets were about the only things happening in Central Florida before Disney and air conditioning. I wasn't interested in orange groves or cattle ranches, but rockets fascinated me and my brother, Alan. While growing up, I read every one of the Tom Swift books about space. These were science fiction books for ten-year old boys similar to the Hardy Boys adventure series or the Nancy Drew mystery series, but these had names like *Tom Swift and His Rocket Ship*, *Tom Swift and His Outpost in Space*, or *Tom Swift and the Race to the Moon*.

Alan and I begged Mom to drive us to Jetty Park right on the Cape whenever a launch was scheduled. Back then, you could get really close, just about two miles away from the launch pad. Sometimes the countdown was stopped in the final minutes, so we never knew what to expect.

Three . . . two . . . one . . . I'll never forget the launch in 1957 when the Vanguard rocket barely rose off the ground, then fell back and blew up in a giant fireball of flame and black smoke. I could practically feel the heat from our vantage point—and the concussive boom of a gigantic rocket blowing up on liftoff.

The newspapers had a field day, calling it *Flopnik* or *Stayputnik* because a few months earlier the Soviet Union had successfully launched Sputnik, which became the first satellite to successfully orbit the Earth, beating us into outer space.

The United States, with national honor on the line, switched to the Juno 1 rocket and put the first successful American satellite into Earth orbit on January 31, 1958, just before midnight. We were there at Cape Canaveral, watching and cheering.

The Space Race was a heady time to be growing up in Central Florida. Pam's father was an aerospace engineer (rocket scientist) who had moved to

Central Florida with the Martin-Marietta Company in 1959. It was a thrilling time to watch the race to put a man on the moon during the 1960s. Pam and I have probably witnessed more than a hundred launches over the years, mostly from our backyard or rooftop because the flame and vapor trails can be seen from the Orlando area.

We've probably witnessed twenty or thirty launches up close, and let me tell you, none were more exciting than watching one of the 363-foot-high Saturn Vs blast off for the moon. Even from a safe distance of more than six miles, the concussive power of the giant booster thumps against your chest. The ground we were standing on would shake, and you could even hear the concussion in Orlando if you listened carefully. That was a thrill of a lifetime.

Then Disney came to Orlando. When they were buying fifty square miles of land to the west of Orlando, the Disney people did it without telling anyone, but toward the end everyone knew something was going on. The common theory in the newspapers was everything was kept under wraps because it had something to do with a top-secret space program or maybe a bombing range. The land was too swampy for cattle or oranges, so what else could it be—maybe a toxic waste dump?

But Walt Disney World opened in 1971, and that story is well known. What's less appreciated is that Disney and the NASA space program produced a certain feeling in those of us who grew up in the Orlando area. That feeling was expressed in the popular song, *If You Can Dream It, You Can Do It*. Everyone who grew up in Central Florida during my generation shares that belief because we've seen it happen.

So with helping those with osteoporosis, I figured that the word might spread faster if a company could be convinced to make a nutritional product that matched the best information available about bone health. Sure, it was a long shot, but least that would help Pam and Sue clear some of the vitamin bottles off their countertops.

Until a commercial business got behind this, I figured I could at least educate other orthopedic surgeons whenever possible. That would be like walking a tight rope, however, because it takes years of solid research to build the trust of academic physicians who want proof and publications. That trust and credibility could disappear with a single false claim, and I'd seen that happen to colleagues in the later stages of their careers.

My documentation had to be complete, balanced, and transparent. I redoubled my efforts and read again all the papers and textbooks—just to make sure nothing had been misinterpreted in any of the data.

The First Steps

My expertise in bone graft substitutes generated invitations on the orthopedic "lecture circuit." Also, the information about silicon in artificial bone grafts was new and interesting to most audiences. That gave me the opportunity to start talking about other aspects of silicon and bone health as part of my lectures on bone graft alternatives.

At the International Pediatric Orthopedic Symposium in December 2007, I had given a lecture in my area of expertise titled "Bone Graft Substitutes," which was well received. That lecture was actually presented a few hours before my mother fell and broke her hip, and it was also presented before silicon-substituted bone grafts were available, so there was no mention of silicon. The very next year, I was invited to give an update on bone graft substitutes, and this time I had new information about silicon-substituted bone grafts.

This was also my first opportunity to talk about bone health, so my talk transitioned right into that topic and kept going. When I added the information about nutrition, the doctors in the audience didn't seem to mind, especially when they learned that beer is good for your bones. They thought that nugget of information was wonderful. Since I was talking about nutrition, I was also judging the reaction of colleagues and registrants to see if they thought I was crazy to wander off the topic of surgery, especially because the symposium was for a group of surgeons.

Several colleagues came up afterwards and wanted to know more. The message had hit home with them, and I had plenty of scientific research to back it up. By that time, I had already learned there was a lot more to bone health than silicon.

A few months after the International Pediatric Orthopedic Symposium, I was asked to speak at a national meeting about spinal fusion surgery in New York City. After presenting my research on bone graft substitutes using human cadaver bone and bone marrow, I talked about the new information from other countries where silicon was incorporated into the artificial bone graft. Again, I transitioned into a discussion of silicon as a nutritional supplement for bone health so they would start thinking that there's more to bone health than calcium and vitamin D.

Once again, my orthopedic colleagues greeted the information about silicon with interest and encouragement. I can't tell you what it meant to receive peer-to-peer confirmation that silicon could be useful to people suffering from declining bone health. That encouraged me to stay at bat and keep swinging.

I drafted a review paper on silicon and osteoporosis and showed it to two orthopedic doctors who routinely publish research papers. These experts were both intrigued by the conclusions and said they would be interested in learning more. They also gave some good feedback about how to spread the word.

You could say that that I was becoming an evangelist for silicon as well as other nutrients that play a role in improving bone mineral density—magnesium, arginine, inositol, boron, and vitamin K.

I got to work on the publication side, wrote two review papers, and submitted them for consideration by widely distributed journals. The first one was titled, "Silicon: A review of its potential role in the prevention and treatment of post-menopausal osteoporosis," and the second was a broader view entitled, "Essential nutrients for bone health with a review of their availability in the typical North American diet."

Both went through a blinded peer review process and were accepted for publication with favorable comments like, "This manuscript is a high quality, well-researched review outlining the important findings while highlighting the unknown facts in a very well balanced way." Another reviewer said, "The subject you have explored is both timely and worthwhile." That was more encouragement.

By this time, I had compiled a formulation for a nutritional supplement to support bone health with silicon, L-arginine, inositol, boron, magnesium, and vitamin K in addition to vitamin D, calcium, and magnesium. I felt there was a real opportunity to produce a product that could help millions facing declining bone health, which was pretty much everyone over the age of fifty-five. That's a *huge* market, as they say in corporate boardrooms. Certainly, there was that at least one nutritional supplement company that would be interested enough to bring this idea to market.

Where do I start looking for someone to take up the banner for a unique nutritional supplement? Well, I had done some consulting work for EBI, a subsidiary of Biomet, by helping them design some spinal surgery instruments and implants that made scoliosis surgery easier. We had also worked together on some bone healing products because EBI, which stood for Electro Biology, Inc., was a leader in implantable technologies, electromagnetic stimulation of bone growth, and some of the traditional bone graft substitutes.

In June 2009, I picked up the phone and had a conversation with the chief of biological research, a Ph.D. in their biological bone-healing research group. We discussed silicon as part of an oral supplement that EBI could develop to help patients heal faster and also to help people with brittle bones from osteoporosis.

I even offered to give him my formulations and all my background research without any legal protection because this was something that might help a lot of people. To some extent, that shows how green I was at the time, but my desire was to get doctors thinking about bone health supplements for osteoporosis as well as something that might help patients recover faster from orthopedic surgery.

The research director listened politely and said that while the concept certainly sounded like it had merit, an oral product didn't fit their corporate business profile or their expertise. He was correct, of course, because EBI did not have a line of nutritional supplements or a pharmaceuticals division, but at least I had some confirmation from another person who knew a lot about basic bone biology.

Okay . . . what was the next step? How about one of the Big Pharma companies—a multinational corporation with billions of dollars in capital that would easily have the resources to introduce a silicon-based product to the masses? I noodled around the websites of several major pharmaceutical companies, especially the ones with over-the-counter multivitamins and brands that included calcium and vitamin D for bone health.

The websites were helpful, but hinted that they were overrun with suggestions for nutritional supplements that made claims for all sorts of miracle cures. I learned that anyone approaching these companies with a product idea needed to have a patent first. That was probably their way of making sure the idea had merit.

I didn't have a patent for my formulations, but it sounded like a good idea to get a professional search of the field, especially if that would help gain entry to a drug company. I hired a patent attorney and a patent agent who researched whether a similar patent had already been filed by someone else. Finding nothing, they successfully applied for a formulation patent. My primary intention was to improve my credibility with these drug companies, some of whom had hired me as a product development consultant in the past.

It took a few months to go through the process of filing for a patent and making sure that nothing else was similar. Then, even with a patent in hand, I never got to first base with the major pharmaceutical companies, but that wasn't a big shock.

Listen, I have the greatest respect for these companies. They are often demonized by the media, but we live much longer, happier, and healthier lives because of their work. It seemed like my idea was small potatoes for them, so it was time to look elsewhere. At least now I had a patent, and I was also learning a lot about how the world worked outside of the operating room.

Perhaps these stumbling efforts seem foolish or naive in retrospect, but the production and marketing of something nutritional was unfamiliar territory. All I wanted to do was find someone who could move the process along a little faster. From my experience, I knew that it usually took five to ten years for information to move from "bench to bedside," a common medical phrase meaning from the research bench to patient care, and that was too slow for my preferences.

So, what was the next step now?

Like everyone else, I'd seen the large chain stores for nutritional health. Perhaps one of those would develop a product—using my patented formulation. Perhaps they could be convinced to make and market a product for those who needed something extra for bone health—something that would make up for insufficiencies in the typical American diet and still allow people to take their daily multivitamin and omega-3.

I sent a letter to GNC—General Nutrition Centers, a national retail chain—in June 2010. That letter included my curriculum vitae (academic résumé) so they might take me seriously. The letter told them about the concept that I wanted to discuss with them. This sentence was even included in the letter: "If you have a product like this that I don't know about, or you're developing a product similar to mine, I would like to help you promote it. I just want to get the word out."

This time I singled and reached first base. The chief innovation officer, a Ph.D. who could understand the science, contacted me. He listened patiently and said he would give my idea serious consideration. We had several conversations, including one in which he informed me that they were so intrigued by the information that they considered developing this as their first internally produced supplement. At the end of the day, however, their company was more of a distributor and not a developer or manufacturer of nutritional supplements.

That was both good news and bad news. The idea was good, but I was looking in the wrong place. At the end of our last conversation, the GNC chief innovation officer referred me to one of their biggest manufacturers and said I could use his name as a reference. Perhaps they could help me, he said.

I did some more research about this other company, and I liked his recommendation. They had experience with bone health and had a good reputation for quality. They had even supported research on some of their products to make sure their products were effective. The products they were offering for bone health had some of the nutrients that were important, but a little tweaking might make a big difference.

I sent a letter to the president and CEO that was similar to the one I'd sent to GNC. All of my contact information was in the correspondence, in addition to my curriculum vitae and an outline of the concept. A response came by email about a week later, informing me that the company had been sold and was being consolidated with a larger manufacturing company located in Florida.

By now it was December 2010, and I had been trying for almost eight months to find someone who would produce a supplement that didn't currently exist for bone health. I was beginning to think that this wasn't going to happen. Hundreds of hours had been spent getting up to speed, then more time grinding away at loads of information. By now, I had increased the size and scope of my home library and paid for patent work, but none of that had opened any doors.

The last email gave me the name of the new manufacturing company in Florida, but it didn't include an introduction or the name of the CEO. The company in Florida was private, making it very difficult to find the name of the corporate executives, much less the CEO himself. After some investigation, I did find the CEO's name and also learned that they had previously produced a product that had some potential for bone health, but that product was no longer being manufactured.

I doubted that another email or letter would go anywhere. It seemed like this company had plenty of business and probably wasn't looking for any new products, especially one that might replace one of the supplements they were already selling. From their perspective they would be taking a chance, especially when their somewhat similar product had already been taken off the shelves because of poor sales.

Well, I'd come this far, so it didn't seem like much more effort to contact this company. I penned my last letter, attached my curriculum vitae one more time, and put it in the mail to the CEO of the manufacturing company in Florida.

As I went to the post office and slipped the letter in the slot, I told myself that this was the last gasp. If my inquiry was met with silence, then I planned to give up. Besides, I still had academic circles where I could keep talking until someone else picked up the banner and carried it forward. If something happened, then it was supposed to happen.

Christmas came and went, and nothing came back by email or mail. In January, I taught a month-long course at the University of Central Florida medical school. By February, I had mentally moved on, although I continued to include more nutritional information in my lectures to the second-year medical students. They lapped it up and wanted more.

Then in early February, a woman named Pam McWilliams emailed me out of the blue and introduced herself as the director of new product development at a high-quality nutritional supplement company in New York. She gave me the name of the company in her email, but I had never heard of it.

Why she contacted me was initially confusing to me because this wasn't the company that had received my letter. She explained that my letter to the president of the new company in Florida had landed on her desk after a two-month journey because her company was a subsidiary of the one in Florida. For some reason, Pam McWilliams wanted to speak with me directly on the phone. I had no clue whether she was going to tell me to move on or that her company had some interest. I knew nothing about the division she worked for.

Pam McWilliams said the reason for her phone call was to inform me that she was quite intrigued by my idea and wanted to hear more. After so much indifference and rejection from other companies, I was overjoyed to hear of her personal interest. In fact, we clicked on the phone that day. She sounded like she was genuinely interested in what I was trying to do, and her interest was for all the right reasons. It was an amazing feeling to hear someone say that my idea might help people. *She got it.*

I didn't want to miss this opportunity, so I offered to take a plane to New York City and meet with her in person. A week later, I flew into JFK and grabbed a rental car for the drive to her office an hour north of Manhattan. The company offices were located in a wooded business park that was a bit hard to find. Once I arrived, she showed me around, and it was obvious that people loved working with her. Then we met in a small conference room where I presented my story about silicon, what the formulations entailed, the science behind these nutrients, and what they might do for people with low bone mineral density.

Then I blew out a breath of air and sat back, waiting for her response. Quite frankly, if Pam McWilliams had said, *thanks but no thanks*, then I was finished for certain. Instead, she said she liked the idea for a silicon-based supplement and that she wanted to champion this concept with her company. Her encouragement meant the world to me since this was the most cheering I'd heard in the last year. Finally, it seemed like something good was going to happen.

We parted with promises to stay in touch and see where the idea went with her company. But then another blow came just a few weeks later when Pam McWilliams informed me that her division was being re-located to Florida and she had decided to stay in New York. She said because of her family, she would not be making the move to Florida, meaning she would be leaving the company.

I admired her decision because she had a good career and future in Florida, but her priorities lay with her family in New York. At the same time, though, it was clear that I was losing an advocate.

Even though she was leaving the company, Pam McWilliams continued to be my biggest booster and didn't want me to give up. She encouraged me to visit the new management in Florida and press my case with them. With her encouragement ringing in my ears, I soldiered on.

My attorney and I drove down Interstate 95 to meet with the new product development people, and the reaction was positive. They said they would get back to us.

But nothing happened. After a couple of months passed by, it became apparent that the idea had "died in committee," as they say.

I phoned New York to talk with Pam McWilliams again and see if she had heard anything through her grapevine. She extended her regrets that things didn't work out, but informed me that she had decided to strike off on her own as a freelance consultant. She encouraged me not to give up. "Your idea is too good," she said.

Before we signed off, Pam McWilliams mentioned that she was going to South Florida for a conference being hosted by one her clients, Jordan Rubin, the founder of a new company called Beyond Organic that was producing grass-fed beef that was "beyond" the USDA standards for organic beef.

Hearing that she would be in my home state, I wanted to ask her in person whether I should give up or keep going. Perhaps there were other supplement suppliers that weren't going through corporate restructuring and buy-outs. Maybe there were some smaller companies that would want to help develop a new product. Or maybe people were giving me lip service and putting my letters in the round file (trash can) for a reason.

I knew I'd get a straight answer even if it wasn't what I wanted to hear. Pam McWilliams had a caring personality but a no-nonsense approach. When I asked if we could meet for lunch when she was in Florida, she said yes.

Also, another notion was beginning to emerge, and that was the notion of starting my own company. This might be the only way to get a different nutritional supplement out there.

I had a feeling that Pam McWilliams was just the right person to hear me out.

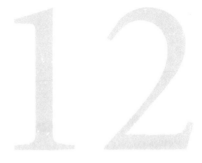

Launching into the Great Unknown

It was an idea that had been rumbling in my mind that I couldn't ignore: *Maybe I'll have to start a company to make this happen.* I must confess that this was a frightening thought and not my original intention. But it was definitely my sub-conscious speaking.

The first few times that idea popped into my head, I dismissed it as being far-fetched and unrealistic. What did I, a pediatric orthopedic surgeon for the last thirty-four years, know about starting or running a nutritional supplement business?

The answer was next to nothing. Actually, that wasn't true. I had learned a few things about the business while pursuing the idea of finding a pharmaceutical or nutritional company to take on a new product.

To meet Pam McWilliams in Ft. Lauderdale, I drove south four hours along Florida's spine, down the Florida Turnpike, which was called the Sunshine State Parkway when it was first built. By this time in our professional relationship, I trusted Pam McWilliams to give me the unvarnished truth.

Over a lunch of black bean soup at a Cuban restaurant near the West Palm Beach Convention Center, she listened to me lay everything out on the table. About introducing a different product to support bone health. About the opportunity to develop products that might help recovery from spine fusions and broken bones. About finding a someone to help produce and distribute a new product. About how there was a lot more to this nutrition thing than most physicians had time to explore and develop.

After a long discussion, I asked her about the risk involved in investing a chunk of the nest egg that my wife, Pam, and I had put aside for our retirement. This was the first time words like that came out of my mouth about starting a company from thin air.

Instead of dismissing the idea of launching a new company, Pam McWilliams thought the concept had enough merit to bring in some pros— talented marketing people with a long history in the nutritional products industry who could render their opinion. In fact, just the right people happened to be in town: The founding partners of the consulting group McNeely Brewster. Pam McWilliams said they knew the nutritional supplement business forewards and backwards. I didn't know them, but I trusted Pam.

She offered to call them up and see if we could have an impromptu meeting. They were amenable. After lunch, we met them in the lobby of their hotel. Pam introduced me to "Dr. Price" without any other explanation. As far as they were concerned, I could have purchased a mail-order license on the Internet. But they knew Pam, and they trusted her.

We sat and talked for an hour. I held nothing back. "Here it is, guys,"

I said. "If you want to do this—help me develop this product—then let me know where we go from here."

To my amazement, they said they could offer guidance in setting up a new company. We shook on it and rolled up our sleeves.

Starting a business would be a huge departure from everything I'd done in my life up to this point. My wife Pam's expertise in law had allowed me to totally focus on taking care of patients and be involved in academic medicine. As a salaried physician and faculty member in a teaching program, I had enjoyed seeing anyone who walked through the door without worrying about their ability to pay.

My wife took care of everything financial. She guided all of our major purchases, investments, and retirement planning. Pam was good at this and had plenty of experience as a trustee for some large estates, too. That was another blessing for me because most doctors have to do this for themselves when they really are more interested in their patients.

Now, I needed my lawyer-wife's advice more than ever, especially because my previous investment suggestions were usually met with one of two responses from her: "That doesn't make any sense." or "That's not a *bad* idea." I thought that forming a nutritional supplement company was actually a *good* idea, and it was in a field that I did know something about.

I'd also learned a lot and had a pretty good handle on what would be needed, but before presenting a business plan to my lawyer-wife, I needed to think it through a little more. I turned to my adult son, Travis, who has a lot of common sense and would be a good sounding board. After I explained everything to Travis, he said that starting my own nutritional company would be quite an undertaking, but quickly added, "It sounds like you've covered the bases. See what Mom thinks."

That's exactly what I did over the next few days. We discussed everything that I'd learned. My wife put on her lawyer hat and asked a lot of good questions, but after hearing my answers and asking more follow-up questions, she said we should do it and that she would help. I immediately contacted Pam McWilliams, who set up a two-day assessment and planning session in Orlando that included the group from McNeely Brewster.

That planning meeting happened two weeks later because Pam McWilliams didn't mess around. When we were finished with the two-day review, the team at McNeely Brewster went to work and conducted a "needs assessment" as well as a "market assessment" that critically looked at the viability of a silicon-based nutritional supplement. Then they, along with Pam MicWilliams, put together a business plan, cash-flow projections, timetables, and a pro forma that could be used to approach investors.

At this point, other investors were needed. I wanted to team up with orthopedic surgeons who understood the science behind the bones. We needed talented and respected physicians who were knowledgeable about good bone health; colleagues who would speak the truth to me and others. That meant orthopedic surgeons who had dedicated their careers to helping patients. The culture of this business would be to promote bone and joint health through improved nutrition.

Four doctors immediately came to mind. Three were part of our teaching program, and the fourth was going to join us in a few months. Each has dedicated his career to the advancement of orthopedic surgery through teaching, writing, and opening their practices to full-time education of residents and fellows.

As expected, they wanted to know a lot more about the science than the business plan, but once they reviewed the science, they were in full support. We decided to call our company the Institute for Better Bone Health and use a direct-to-consumer business model for providing nutritional supplements and educational products to those seeking to strengthen their bones in middle age and beyond. The four colleagues were also four friends, and each one was enthusiastic about the project.

My four partners are:

• **Kenneth J. Koval, M.D.,** who recently joined us from Dartmouth Medical School, where he was a Professor of Orthopedic Surgery. In addition to his other accomplishments, Ken is widely recognized as one of the world's leading authorities on broken hips, having published two books and several textbook chapters on hip fractures.

In addition, he has published more than 150 peer-reviewed scientific articles about hip fractures, including predictors of mortality, frequency, geographic variations, geriatric treatment, biomechanics, fixation methods, bone graft substitutes, bone growth proteins, and other adjuncts to improve fracture healing. He also serves on editorial boards of several prestigious journals.

All that work has been done without any financial compensation—no money, nada—because that's what academic orthopedic surgeons do . . . give their knowledge and expertise for the good of the profession and for the good of the public.

Ken is also a scientific skeptic whom I could count on to read all the data and look at the original research to satisfy himself that everything was on the level.

• **George Haidukewych, M.D.,** is Chairman of the Orthopedic Residency Program and Chief of the Orthopedic Surgery Practice at Orlando Health. He is also a Professor of Orthopaedic Surgery at the University of Central Florida. Clinically, Dr. Haidukewych is a fellowship-trained trauma surgeon and co-director of the Orthopaedic Trauma Service at Orlando Health. He is also Chief of Complex Adult Reconstruction. In addition to his trauma duties, he has performed a significant number of complex revision total joint cases. His practice also includes post-traumatic reconstructive surgery of the hip and knee joint, as well as management of serious infections.

Dr. Haidukewych received his M.D. degree from Wayne State University School of Medicine in Detroit, Michigan, where he was valedictorian of his medical school class. He then completed his residency at the Mayo Clinic in Rochester, Minnesota. After his trauma fellowship in Tampa, Florida, he returned to the Mayo Clinic where he served as Chief of Orthopaedic Trauma. He then joined the Florida Orthopaedic Institute in Tampa, where he served as co-director of the Adult Reconstructive Fellowship and Associate Professor at the University of South Florida.

Dr. Haidukewych has authored over forty scientific research studies, including aspects of hip and knee joint replacement, treatment of non-unions, computer-assisted surgery, and fracture management. He has also served as a reviewer for several orthopedic journals and published several chapters in orthopedic textbooks. While on the faculty at the Mayo Clinic, Dr. Haidukewych was the Director of Orthopedic Basic Science Education and was recognized as Teacher of the Year by the orthopedic residents.

George has excellent business judgment and helps oversee the finances of our company.

• **Joshua Langford, M.D.,** was born and raised in rural northern Illinois. He attended Washington University in St. Louis for his undergraduate degree and then continued on to the University of Illinois College of Medicine for his medical degree. Then he completed the Orthopedic Surgery Residency Program at Mount Sinai Hospital in New York, followed by an orthopedic trauma fellowship at Tampa General Hospital. His special interests included limb lengthening, limb salvage, bone infection, and pelvic fractures.

Josh has made numerous scientific presentations nationally and internationally and has published several papers in peer-reviewed journals. He is a reviewer for the *Journal of Orthopaedic Trauma* as well as *Clinical Orthopaedics and Related Research*. He has been deeply involved in resident and fellow education and continues to be involved in ongoing research related to orthopaedic trauma. He has volunteered his surgical skills in Ethiopia, Peru, India, and the Dominican Republic.

Dr. Langford has special training and expertise in computer-assisted surgery for trauma and limb deformity surgery, including limb lengthening. Josh is also very knowledgeable about nutritional supplements.

• **Frank Liporace, M.D.**, is a highly regarded orthopedic trauma physician who has brought innovation to his field. He received his medical degree from New York Medical College and completed his orthopedic surgery training at NYU Hospital for Joint Diseases Orthopaedic Institute in New York City. After that, Frank completed an orthopedic trauma fellowship in Tampa, Florida. He then joined the faculty at the University of Medicine and Dentistry of New Jersey, where he rose rapidly to the rank of Associate Professor.

Frank specializes in the treatment of complex fractures, including fractures that involve the joints or go through the joint surfaces. The other major part of his practice is joint replacement surgery, including difficult revision cases and patients with osteoporosis. Moreover, Frank has published some high-quality research with over forty manuscripts, numerous book chapters, and over 200 lectures nationally and internationally.

Before Frank joined our group in Orlando, I had heard him deliver an outstanding presentation about bone graft substitutes and the biology of bone healing. I knew then that Frank understood bone health in a way that would help our effort. Better yet, Frank has a rare combination of good business sense, clinical excellence, intellectual curiosity, and an understanding of basic bone biology.

This group of four orthopedic surgeons all saw the benefits down the road for helping bones grow stronger and for helping bone healing. It's especially nice to have people you can trust and rely on to help you make decisions about what goes into the product. They also understood the need to spend some of any profits on research to improve bone health.

Better Bone Health Now

At this point, we had everything needed to get started: good intentions, experienced consultants, a group of dedicated physicians, and a patented product that showed a lot of potential to improve bone health. Our group of doctors had several heart-to-heart meetings where we talked about the financial risk of starting a new business. The task was daunting to a group of academic orthopedic surgeons.

We dove deep into the science of the proposed product for general bone health. We discussed some other potentially beneficial products that might come from such a venture. Once we started thinking about the impact that nutrition could have on the entire practice of orthopedic surgery, we knew this company was something we had to do.

After lengthy discussions and more research, we came up with an additional product that may help natural bone healing after a broken bone or after orthopedic surgery. That's exciting stuff because each of us had been asked hundreds of times by our patients whether there was anything they could take to help their bones heal better. Until now, our answer had always been the same: "Just eat healthy and increase your dairy intake a little." Now that our eyes were opened, we knew there was a lot more that might be possible.

We officially formed the Institute for Better Bone Health so that we could produce and sell these products that weren't available anywhere else. Most of all, we wanted to improve bone health now, not ten years from now.

We have developed two products. Our first product is intended to help maintain bone health. We named our first product to emphasize that silicon has an important role in calcification of bone. This product also included the other nutrients that are commonly insufficient, but only in the amounts that would supplement the average American diet, and not megadoses. The purpose was to provide nutrients for bone health because this is what had helped my wife, Pam.

We put the ingredients for the first product in two different bottles because some of the nutrients are taken in the morning and some later in the day or at night. The reason we did this is because pills that combine everything may cause competition for absorption in the digestive tract. Few other products have recognized this important aspect of bone health.

The second product is intended to be used for shorter periods of time to support natural bone repair after trauma or surgery. This one is supposed to be used with the first product when slightly larger doses and some extra ingredients might be needed. Once the increased needs have passed, then the first product for bone maintenance should be enough for long-term bone support.

We Have Liftoff

Time will tell whether this will be successful or not. This group of doctors is risking a great deal of financial resources to launch a new company in a less-than-ideal economic climate. Where will this effort take us?

The quick answer is, "I don't know," but we do have the right group of people on board. My partners have dedicated their careers to helping others, and it shows in their work. My wife, Pam, has never wavered from her commitment that "we should do some things to help people."

So, we'll see what happens with the Institute for Better Bone Health, but we'll be okay if we stick to our core principles and don't get sidetracked from our purpose of improving bone health and trying to help doctors help their patients.

I think Mom would have approved.

Part II

Additional Information About Bone Health

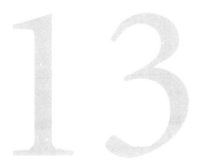

Nutrition Summary

Dietary Supplements for Bone Health

Proper nutrition is one component of good bone health. When diet alone cannot provide adequate nutrition, then supplementation is a reasonable choice. Children's vitamins often have enough of the everyday nutrients for adults who consume a typical American diet.

All foods have some nutrients, so a little supplementation without megadoses can usually satisfy the general health needs of adults. When there are specific concerns like poor bone health, then some extra supplementation may be helpful. For general health and for bone health, it's probably helpful to take three additional supplements.

1. Daily omega-3 fish oil—good for general health and better than the same amount of flaxseed oil.

2. Daily multivitamin:

   o Children's vitamins often have enough of the B vitamins and other nutrients for general health.

   o Preferably the multivitamin will have limited amounts of the following for otherwise healthy people:

     • Vitamin A—the beta-carotene type is preferred if in a multivitamin

     • Vitamin E

     • Vitamin B_6

     • Metals:

       Selenium

       Zinc

       Manganese

       Copper

       Strontium

       Iron

3. For bone health, an extra supplement helps reduce the risk of fracture. All of the nutrients listed next have very high upper limits without adverse effects, but too much supplementation with calcium and magnesium can cause higher levels than recommended by the U.S. National Institutes of

Health (NIH).

- Calcium—preferably not more than 1,000 mg/day as a supplement because the tolerable upper level of total intake from diet and supplements is 2,000 mg/day, according to the NIH

- Magnesium—not more than 350 mg/day as a supplement, according to the NIH.

- Vitamin D

- Silicon—the silicon dioxide form is poorly absorbed

- Boron

- Vitamin K

- Inositol

- L-arginine

- Vitamin C

Food Sources of Nutrients for Bone Health

Healthy foods are the best source of nutrients because micronutrients like phytochemicals have biological properties that aren't completely understood. High-salt foods also contribute to calcium loss and osteoporosis. [155]

Here is a list of some known nutrients for bone health, the Recommended Dietary Allowance (RDA), and approximate nutritional content in some common foods. You can see from the foods listed below that some have several essential nutrients for bone health.

Calcium—RDA 1,200 mg/day, but the majority of American women older than forty consume less than 600 mg/day.

o 8 ounces of milk or yogurt	350 mg
o 1.5 ounces cheddar or mozzarella cheese	300 mg
o 1 cup frozen yogurt, cream cheese, or cottage cheese	125 mg
o 6 ounces of calcium-fortified orange juice	375 mg
o 2 ounces of almonds	150 mg
o 3 ounces canned salmon or sardines	200 mg
o ½ cup spinach, kale, bok choy, mustard, or turnip greens	100 mg
o ½ cup broccoli, green beans	20 mg

Magnesium—RDA 320 mg/day, but the majority of American women older than forty consume less than 225 mg/day.

o 2 ounces of almonds or cashews	160 mg
o 2 ounces of peanuts or mixed nuts	100 mg
o 1 cup raisin bran, bran flakes, or shredded wheat cereal	75 mg
o medium baked potato with skin	50 mg
o ½ cup brown rice, black-eyed peas, kidney beans, or lentils	35 mg
o 8 ounces of milk	25 mg

Vitamin D—RDA 600-800 IU, but Endocrine Society recommends 1,500 IU. The majority of American women older than forty consume less than 200 IU/day.

NOTE: It's almost impossible to get enough vitamin D from food sources alone.

o 1 tablespoon cod liver oil	1,350 IU
o 3 ounces swordfish or salmon	500 IU
o 3 ounces canned tuna fish	150 IU
o 8 ounces of vitamin D-fortified milk	125 IU
o 3 ounces beef liver, or one large egg yolk	40 IU

Silicon—RDA not established, increased bone mineral density when more than 40 mg/day. The average dietary intake for women older than fifty is approximately 20 mg/day.

o 16 ounces of beer	12 mg
o 16 ounces mineral water, depending on brand	0-40 mg
o 1 serving of whole-grain breakfast cereal, granola	9 mg
o 3 ounces of raisins	8 mg
o ½ cup brown rice or green beans	4 mg

Boron—RDA not established. Increased bone mineral metabolism when more than 3 mg/day. The average intake of Boron is approximately 1mg/day.

o Small box of raisins, ¼ cup prunes, or almonds   1 mg

o cup of apricots or half an avocado   1 mg

o cup of dry roasted peanuts or hazelnuts   1 mg

Vitamin K—RDA 90 µgm (micrograms)/day for women. Improved bone density is reported with more than 109 µgm/day. Average dietary intake of vitamin K in the U.S. is 80 µgm/day, and more than half the population consumes less than 70 µgm/day. Vitamin K should not be taken with blood thinner Coumadin®, but megadoses do not have adverse effects and do not increase clotting in people who are not taking Coumadin®.

o ½ cup cooked kale or collards   500 µgm

o 1 cup fresh spinach   140 µgm

o ½ cup cooked broccoli or Brussels sprouts   120 µgm

o ½ head iceberg lettuce or ¾ cup raw broccoli   70 µgm

o ½ cup coleslaw or 1 cup blueberries   40 µgm

Inositol—no RDA because the body can make inositol. It is estimated that the body consumes a few grams of inositol each day. Supplementation has been beneficial for some disorders such as polycystic ovaries and panic disorders. Experimental studies have reported improved bone mineral density with inositol supplementation. Inositol from fruits may be more beneficial than inositol from hulls of grains and beans.

o ¼ cantaloupe	355 mg
o 1 fresh orange, 1 slice stone ground whole wheat bread	300 mg
o ¼ cup of prunes (6 to 8 prunes)	250 mg
o ½ fresh grapefruit, or 1 fresh lime	200 mg
o ½ cup green beans	150 mg
o 1 kiwi fruit	130 mg
o 1 cup watermelon, or one fresh peach	60 mg
o 1 cup chocolate milk	45 mg

L-arginine—RDA not established. Average U.S. intake is 4.4 gm/day with one quarter of the population consuming less than 2.6 mg/day. L-arginine helps arteries relax and improves blood flow, but should not be taken after an acute heart attack. Large doses have been taken over periods of several years without harmful effects.

o 3 ounces of chicken, turkey, beef, or pork	2.0 gm
o 3 ounces salmon or shrimp	1.1 gm
o ¼ cup peanuts	1.0 gm
o ¼ cup almonds	0.8 gm

o one whole egg   0.8 gm

o ¼ cup cashew nuts   0.7 gm

Vitamin C—RDA 75 mg/day. Half of all women in the U.S. between the ages of forty and sixty years consume less than 63 mg/day. Megadoses are not recommended, but increased doses of vitamin C have improved bone healing in experimental studies.

o ¾ cup orange juice   93 mg

o ¾ cup grapefruit juice   70 mg

o ½ cup cooked broccoli   51 mg

o ½ cup fresh strawberries   49 mg

o ¾ cup tomato juice   33 mg

o ½ cup cantaloupe   29 mg

o 1 raw medium tomato   17 mg

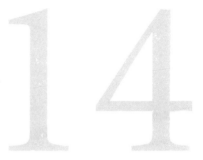

Practical Tips for Bone Health

How Worried Should You Be?

Osteoporosis should be taken seriously because people are living longer and want to enjoy physical health as long as possible. Also, four out of ten Caucasian women over the age of fifty are expected to break a bone unless something is done to reduce the risk of osteoporosis.[10]

The good news is that improvements in bone health are possible for those who are willing to make small changes in their dietary habits and lifestyle. Other good news is that scientific understanding of osteoporosis is increasing rapidly.

Thirty years ago, osteoporosis was often considered a normal part of growing older, and there wasn't much scientific knowledge about osteoporosis. One reason why there is so much attention to osteoporosis today is because simple measures may make big differences.

This section will review some misunderstandings, but it will also try to give perspective to the growing concern with osteoporosis.

Are You at Risk for Osteoporosis?

Everyone over the age of fifty is at risk for osteoporosis, especially thin Caucasian or Asian women, and people with poor health. Even men should be concerned about bone health because one man in eight is at risk for a broken bone after the age of fifty.[10]

You can use the methods in this section to estimate your risk of osteoporosis and your risk of having a broken bone in the future. If your risks are worrisome, then bone density testing can be done to make the predictions more accurate.

■ The Osteoporosis Self-Assessment Score (OST Score)

An easy way to estimate your risk of osteoporosis is called the Osteoporosis Self-Assessment Score (OST Score). The OST is based on age and weight. This calculation was developed to predict the risk of osteoporosis for postmenopausal women. [155, 156] With a slight modification it can be used for men and pre-menopausal women.[157, 158]

Here are the steps:

1. Calculate your weight in kilograms.

   a. If you know your weight in pounds, then divide by 2.2 to determine the number of kilograms you weigh.

2. Subtract your age from your weight in kilograms. The answer may be a negative, or minus, number.

3. Divide by 5. The answer may be a negative number

4. Interpretation for Postmenopausal women

Score worse than -3	High risk of osteoporosis
Score between 1 and -3	Moderate risk of osteoporosis
Score 1 or more	Low risk of osteoporosis

> *Example:* A woman's weight is 130 pounds and her age is 66 years old
>
> 130 lbs divided by 2.2 = 59 Kg
>
> 59 minus 66 = -7
>
> -7 divided by 5 = -1.4 (Moderate risk of osteoporosis)

5. Interpretation for Men and for younger women who are premenopausal women or less than two years post-menopausal

Any score less than 2 means an increased risk of osteoporosis

> *Example:* A woman's weight is 130 pounds and her age is 44 years old
>
> 130 lbs divided by 2.2 = 59 Kg
>
> 59 minus 44 = 15
>
> 15 divided by 5 = 3 (Low risk of osteoporosis)

■ Additional risk factors should be considered when there is moderate risk for osteoporosis. These include:

o History of fracture after the age of 45

o Parent with history of hip fracture

o Tobacco use

o Excessive alcohol use

o Body mass index less than 22 kg/m^2 (see chart on page 123)

o Having a baby before the age of 18

o No children or pregnancies

o Other illnesses

   • Diabetes

   • Inflammatory bowel disease

   • Glucocorticoid (steroids) use more than three months

   • Using Coumadin® blood thinner

BMI is less than 22 kg/m^2 when

Height (inches)	Weight less than (pounds)
58	105
59	109
60	112
61	116
62	120
63	124
64	128
65	132
66	136
67	140
68	144
69	149
70	153
71	157
72	162
73	166
74	171
75	176
76	180

Common medicines and habits that are associated with poor bone health:

o Ibuprofen (Advil) and naproxen (Naprosyn, Aleve)[159]

o long-term use of proton pump inhibitors (e.g. Prilosec, Prevacid, Nexium)[160]

o excessive vitamin A[161]

o cigarettes[10]

o excessive alcohol[10]

Are You at Risk for Fracture?

Having low bone density or osteoporosis doesn't mean that you will have a fracture. There are other factors that affect the risk of fracture. The World Health Organization has developed a calculation tool called FRAX® that is basically a questionnaire.[162, 163]

This calculation tool is available at the following website: http://www.shef.ac.uk/FRAX/. The calculation predicts whether you are at an increased risk for fracture. The calculation tool uses height in centimeters and weight in kilograms, but there is also a weight and height conversion calculator on the website.

If you had a DXA scan, your doctor probably did this calculation for you. The fracture risk calculation may be more accurate when the bone mineral density is known, but it can be used with only the body mass index (BMI) that can be automatically calculated on the FRAX® website. There are also blood tests for bone turnover that may improve the estimation of fracture risk.[164]

FRAX® is considered the standard for calculation of fracture risk, but another test called the Fracture Index was developed before FRAX® to predict fractures for Caucasian women in the United States.[165] This test is self-scored and is shown below in a modified form. The score for each question is determined, and the total score for all questions added together is compared to the graphs to determine the five-year risk of hip fracture and the five-year risk of all fractures combined. If the T-score (see below) is known, the test is a little more reliable.

Fracture Index test: Each answer has a certain number of points. Circle the points for each question and add them up at the end of the test. (*Adapted from*, Black, DM, et.al. An assessment tool for predicting fracture risk in postmenopausal women. *Osteoporosis International* 2001; 12:519-28, and is used with permission.)

1. What is your current age?

Less than 65 years	0 points
65-69 years	1 point
70-75 years	2 points
75-79 years	3 points
80-85 years	4 points
85 and older	5 points

2. Have you broken any bones after age 50?

Yes	1 point
No	0 points

3. Has your mother had a hip fracture after age 50?

Yes	1 point
No	0 points

4. Do you weigh 125 pounds or less?

Yes	1 point
No	0 points

5. Are you currently a smoker?

Yes	1 point
No	0 points

6. Do you usually need to use your arms to assist yourself in standing up from a chair?

Yes	2 points
No	0 points

After adding the points from those six questions, calculate your fracture risk..

Total Points	5-year risk of spine fracture	5-year risk of fracture besides the spine	5-year risk specifically for hip fracture
1	140%	10.50%	0.60%
2	2.90%	12.50%	1.40%
3	5.10%	16.40%	2.10%
4	5.10%	18.70%	3.20%
5 or more	9.90%	26.10%	8.20%

7. If you have had a bone density (BMD) test, then answer the next question and add the points to the total of the other six questions.
   a. T-score -1 or better   0 points
   b. T-score between -1 and -2   2 points
   c. T-score between -2 and -2.5   3 points
   d. T-score worse than – 2.5   4 points

Total Points with BMD points	5-year risk of spine fracture	5-year risk of fracture other than spine	5-year risk specifically for hip fracture
1 or 2	1.20%	8.60%	0.40%
3 or 4	2.50%	13.10%	0.90%
5	5.30%	16.50%	1.90%
6 or 7	7.10%	19.80%	3.90%
8 through 13	11.20%	27.50%	8.70%

Tests for Bone Mineral Density

Bone mineral density is only a measure of how much mineral, mainly calcium, there is in the bones. Bone mineral density is measured on a DXA scan, and this is currently the most reliable test for fracture risk, but the bone mineral density doesn't tell the whole story.[164] There are other properties of bone, such as stiffness and diameter, that are important for strength.[12]

Exercise tends to make bones larger, in addition to improving mineral density. The flexibility of bones may be improved with certain nutrients, such as vitamin K, without changing the bone mineral density.[84]

The shape of the bone can influence the risk of fracture regardless of bone mineral density. An example is that hip fractures are more common in women with a long femoral neck.[166]

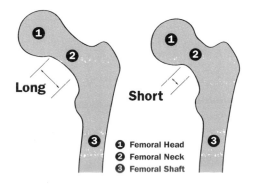

❶ Femoral Head
❷ Femoral Neck
❸ Femoral Shaft

Tests for bone mineral density

○ **X-rays**—bones should be white or light grey on regular x-rays. If they are dark grey with thin margins, then there may be low bone mineral density. The whiter the bone, the denser the bone. Regular X-rays can't usually detect osteoporosis until about half of the bone mineral is gone.

○ **DXA Scan**—this is currently the most important method of testing bone mineral density. This test uses an X-ray method to measure the bone mineral density in your hip and spine. The absolute bone mineral density is measured in grams of mineral per square centimeter of bone, or g/cm^2. That amount is compared to the average bone mineral density of young healthy women to determine the T-score. This is reported as the standard deviation (SD) from the mean (average).[167]

When bone density is equal to the upper 85% of young women, it is considered normal and has a T-score above -1 SD. When the bone mineral density is in the lower 6% to 15% of the young adult population, then the T-score is between -1 and -2.5 SD. This is considered *osteopenia* and means that the bone is thinner than it should be.

When the bone mineral density is in the lowest 6% of the young adult population, then the T-score is worse than -2.5 SD and this is called *osteoporosis*. When a fragility fracture has already occurred and the T-score is worse than -2.5, then the condition is called *established osteoporosis*.

Proportion of Population (%)

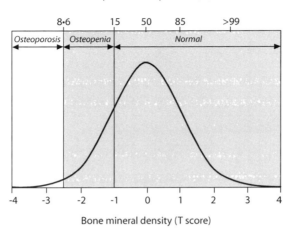

Bone mineral density (T score)

(*From* Kanis, JA. Diagnosis of osteoporosis and assessment of fracture risk. *Lancet* 2002; 359:1929-36; used with permission)

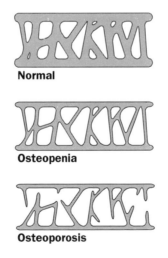

Normal

Osteopenia

Osteoporosis

- **Qualitative ultrasound (QUS) of the calcaneus (heel bone)**—this is an easily performed test that avoids the use of X-rays. QUS measures bone structure and predicts fracture risk independent of bone mineral density.[12, 168]

NOTE: Combining the QUS and DXA scan results may be more accurate to predict fractures than either test alone.[169] Qualitative ultrasound is increasing in popularity, but in 2012 the DXA scan is still recommended as the best test to evaluate osteoporosis.

What Does It Mean to Have Osteopenia or Osteoporosis?

Osteopenia means low bone mineral density but not usually bad enough to need drug treatment. *Osteoporosis* is the medical term that's used to describe a disease state. *Established osteoporosis* means that the disease state is present and has already caused a problem. [167]

Osteopenia, or low bone mineral density, is a warning sign for future broken bones, but it's also a warning sign for possible hunched over posture, bone pain, and limited mobility. This warning sign should be taken seriously, but there's no need to panic if the T-score is in the osteopenic range. There's plenty of evidence that good nutrition and modest exercise during the early stages of bone loss can improve bone health without resorting to prescription medicines.[170]

There are studies showing that vitamin D and calcium supplements can decrease the risk of fractures in women who have never had a fragility fracture.[171, 172] Adding other nutrients, stopping smoking, and exercising may decrease the risk of fracture even more than calcium and vitamin D alone, so it's worthwhile to improve nutrition and exercise as a foundation for bone health.

It may be helpful to understand the true risk of hip fracture and how this risk is reported for those who take medicines. Sixteen percent of women, or one out of six, are predicted to have a hip fracture between the ages of fifty and eighty years.

That's a pretty high risk, but it also means that five out of six won't have a hip fracture.[10] Medicines that produce a 50% decrease in hip fractures sound impressive, but that means the absolute number of hip fractures is half as many as it would have been without the medicine.

For example, suppose 100 women don't take the medicine; then 16 of them would be expected to have a broken hip (16%). Suppose now that 100 other women do take the medicine; then eight of them would be expected to have a broken hip (8%). That means half as many women had a hip fracture if they took the medicine. The true decrease in hip fractures, however, is eight per 100 or an 8% decrease.

Eight percent is a big improvement in the number of hip fractures, but it doesn't sound as impressive as when the drug companies say that their medicine decreases the risk of hip fracture by 50%. It's important to understand this difference so you can evaluate the benefits and risks more accurately. If serious side effects occur in 8% of the people taking a medicine, and the absolute reduction in fractures is 8%, then the risks and benefits may be equal.

This book is written because osteoporosis is a serious problem that affects many women and some men. However, this book is also written to emphasize proper nutrition during early stages of bone loss instead of thinking that drug treatment is inevitable. It's also important to continue good nutrition even when you need prescription medicines for more advanced stages of bone loss.

The National Osteoporosis Foundation has published guidelines for treatment of osteopenia and osteoporosis with prescription medicines. [173] These guidelines recommend medical treatment of a man or woman over the age of fifty in the following circumstances:

1. A hip or vertebral fracture
2. T-score less than or equal to -2.5 after evaluation to exclude other causes

3. Osteopenia (T-score between -1.0 and -2.5) and:

    a. 10-year probability of hip fracture equal to
       or greater than 3%,

    b. or 10-year probability of a major fragility fracture
       of 20% or greater

The first recommendation for treatment is somewhat controversial. That recommendation is intended to apply only to fragility fractures that occur from a fall of less than standing height; not to high-energy injuries like auto accidents that could break strong bones.

Testing for bone mineral density might be worthwhile after any fracture in an older person, but medical treatment of osteoporosis is not needed for every fracture after the age of fifty. The third recommendation is based on osteopenia and the FRAX score that takes into account some of the risk factors, but the final decision may depend on other factors.[164]

Remember that these are guidelines for doctors and not rigid rules for every patient. These guidelines are useful, however, because the benefits of drug treatment generally outweigh the risks when these guidelines are followed for most patients.

Nutrition: a Balanced Approach

This book has been about nutrition and how nutrition can help bone health. Very healthy eating combined with exercise is the best way to maintain bone health. In addition to the proper nutrients, decreasing salt intake is also helpful because high-salt diets are associated with osteoporosis and with hypertension.[155]

When diet alone cannot provide adequate nutrition, then supplementation is a reasonable choice. Vitamin D is a good example of something that needs supplementation for almost everyone, even if they are eating a very healthy diet.

The best approach is a balanced approach without megadoses of any factor. Taking too much of one nutrient is rarely helpful and may be harmful. An exception is Vitamin K_2 that has been used in Japan in megadoses, but even that had a ceiling effect at 45 mg/day.[82]

Studies showed that giving 90 mg/day or 135 mg/day did not reduce fractures more than 45 mg/day. These large doses of vitamin K_2 are called pharmaceutical doses and should be used under the supervision of a physician in the same way as prescription drugs are used.

If you have osteopenia, then nutrition and exercise may help prevent bone loss. Good nutrition is also important when there is established osteoporosis. Those who have experienced a broken bone should do all they can to recover completely, and that often includes good diet, nutritional supplements, exercise, and prescription medications.

Tips for an Exercise Program You Can Do

Exercise is as important as good nutrition. Physical therapists are fond of saying, *If it's physical, it's therapy*. There's a lot of truth to that statement. Exercise improves bone strength, and it also improves flexibility, balance, and muscle strength. So, it's more than just bone strength because exercise can decrease the risk of falls by 25%.[12]

Just fifteen minutes of modest exercise every day, or one hour of exercise twice a week, makes a big difference for health. [174] There's no need to overdose on exercise, unless you want to exercise more for personal enjoyment.

Modest exercise is all that's needed to maintain health. Modest exercise also improves brain function, reduces stress, and decreases the risk of heart attack. Excessive exercise with low body weight actually increases the risk of osteoporosis and fractures.[12]

Exercise programs should strive to improve balance, flexibility, muscle strength, bone strength, and endurance. Before beginning an exercise program on your own, you should probably check with your doctor to make sure your bones, muscles and balance are good enough to attempt some of these exercises without supervision or assistance.

Balance: A simple test of balance for fall prevention is to see if you can do the following: get up from a standard chair without using your arms; walk forward several steps; turn around and walk back to the chair: sit without using your arms. If this can be done easily, then balance is not a problem.[12] There are some simple exercises that may improve balance, but supervision and assistance is recommended, preferably with a physical therapist, unless you already have good balance. Otherwise, simple exercises can begin while holding onto a chair or hand rail.

• Practice standing on one foot at a time for 30 seconds

    Beginners: Raise one leg, bend the knee and hold it still

      o Straighten the raised leg and swing it out to the side or in circles

    For more advanced balance training:

      o lift a weight in one arm held out to the side

      o stand on a sofa pillow

• Walk on tip toes , then heels, and walk sideways for practice

• Tai Chi

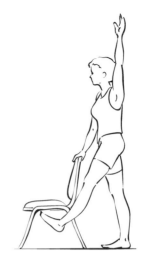

Balance Exercise
A simple balance exercise is to stand on one leg and swing the opposite leg in a circle, or raise and move the arm. Holding onto a chair is safer until balance improves.

Flexibility: Flexibility can be improved by gradual stretching that is held for at least 30 seconds at a time. This allows the muscle to relax and increase length gradually. Stretches can be done while standing, sitting, or while lying on the floor. Some major leg muscles that need to be stretched are the calf muscle, the front and back thigh muscles (quadriceps and hamstrings), and the groin muscles.

• Calf muscle stretch:

  o Sit with the legs out straight and place a towel around the forefoot. Pull the towel toward you while keeping the knees straight. This also strengthens the arms and back.

  o Or place hands on a wall with arms straight. Then keep the feet flat on the floor and back the feet away from the wall while keeping the body as straight as possible. For beginners, do one leg at a time.

• Quadriceps stretch: Stand or lie on one side and grab one foot behind your back with the knee bent. Then press the foot against the buttocks and pull the knee backwards.

• Hamstring stretch:

  ○ Sit with the legs out straight and bend forward at the waist.

  ○ Or stand and put one leg straight out on a chair and bend forward at the waist.

• Groin stretch: sit with the knees bent with the feet touching each other and pulled towards the crotch, then press the knees out to the side to spread the thighs apart.

• Yoga is a bigger commitment, but can improve flexibility.

Muscle strength: Bones get stronger when muscles are stronger. Training with heavier weights and fewer lifts strengthen bone more than lighter weights that are lifted many times.[175] That difference isn't as important as just doing something to improve strength. Some simple exercises for strength and balance can be accomplished without using weights:

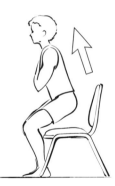

• Slowly rise from a chair and slowly sit down again ten times without using your arms.

  ○ For arm strengthening, repeat this using your arms to push up and to let yourself back down into the chair.

• Lunges are an excellent exercise. Make a large step forward with one leg, then bend the knee of the back leg until it almost touches the floor, then stand up and repeat with the opposite leg. This strengthens the muscles on the front and back of the thigh. Repeat both legs ten times.

- Lie on stomach and lift legs and shoulders off the floor at the same time. Hole ten seconds and repeat ten times. This strengthens the buttocks and spine.

- Lie on your side and lift one leg away from the floor as high as possible. Hold it for ten seconds and repeat ten times. Switch to the other side for the opposite leg.

- Stand and gradually rise up on your toes as high as possible. Let yourself down slowly. Repeat ten times, then rest and repeat another ten times. Hold onto a chair if your balance is poor.

- Lie on your back and bend your knees with the feet on the ground. Fold your arms on your chest and lift your shoulders off the floor. Hold for ten seconds and repeat ten times.

Bone strength: Impact exercises are better than low-impact exercises for building bone density, but swimming has an undeserved bad reputation for osteoporosis.[176] Any type of exercise that requires muscles to act on the bones helps maintain bone strength. A study of senior women swimmers in Australia showed that swimming was effective for maintaining bone mineral density.[177]

Low-impact activities or whole body vibration (see below) should be considered for people with established osteoporosis because impact training can be risky for brittle bones. Some simple impact exercises for bone strengthening are:

- Heel drop—rise up on the tips of your toes and keep the knees straight, then suddenly relax the ankles so the heel strikes the floor with the weight of your body. Repeat 60 times.[178]

• Vertical jump—jump in place with both feet and land firmly. Repeat 30 times.

• Jump training—step onto a low platform of approximately five-to-ten inches and jump down. Repeat 60 times.

• Jumping jacks

Heel Drop Exercise
This is used when the spine is strong enough to withstand some impact. drop—rise up on the tips of your toes and keep the knees straight, then suddenly relax the ankles so the heel strikes the floor with the weight of your body. Begin with only a little impact and gradually increase the force as tolerated.

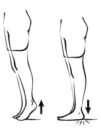

Stair-Stepping Exercise
Stepping up and down builds strength in the calf and thigh muscles. This can be combined with the heel drop if the spine is strong enough and balance is not a big problem. Begin slowly and hold onto a rail or wall until balance, strength, and bone quality permit greater effort and impact.

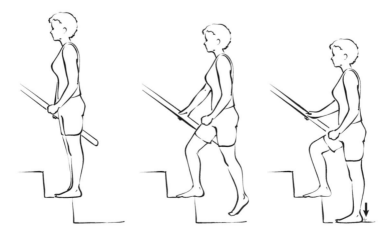

Endurance is good for general health and to improve all aspects of bone health. Activities that require at least fifteen minutes of sustained modest exercise and include balance, light impact, and strengthening are recommended. These include:

- walking

- dancing

- tennis

- exercise classes

Putting together an exercise program. Remember, if it's physical, it's therapy, so don't worry too much about choosing a perfect exercise program. It's more important to get started and spend at least two hours a week exercising. If you prefer fifteen-to-twenty minutes a day, then alternate two programs with one day emphasizing balance, flexibility and strength, while the next day uses the other program to improve bone strength and endurance.

Vibration Therapy

Whole body vibration (WBV) is increasingly popular as a method of exercise training. Experimental studies have shown that vibration increases bone formation and bone mineral density. [179-182]WBV is being used in physical therapy, rehabilitation, and professional sports.

Currently, there are many different types of vibration platforms and different recommendations for use, but there is no specific protocol for osteoporosis, and this method is not recognized by the FDA as a treatment for osteoporosis.[179] There is a promising field of research, however, that may show benefits for bone health in the near future.

Low-intensity WBV may be more easily tolerated by older adults, and there is some evidence that this may improve balance along with improved muscle and bone health.[180] Whole body vibration machines are generally about the size of weighing scales in a doctor's office. The person stands or sits on a vibrating platform and can hold onto the handle bars attached to the upright portion of the machine. One study in postmenopausal women reported increased bone mineral density in the vertebrae after fifteen minutes of daily vibration therapy for one year.[183]

Whole body vibration therapy also has positive effects on muscle function, but possible adverse effects are not fully known.[179] Adverse effects may include falling from the platform, blurry vision, and possible effects on internal organs. In spite of these concerns, whole body vibration may be especially useful for people who are too feeble to walk.

Tips for Home Safety and Fall Prevention

Exercise and nutrition are important for prevention of falls, and vitamin D has a beneficial effect on muscle as well as on bone. Numerous studies have noted improvement in balance, muscle strength, and coordination with increasing levels of vitamin D supplementation.[184]

In contrast, bisphosphonates improve bone mineral density without helping muscle function. Boron has also been shown to improve balance and coordination. Adequate intake of these and other nutrients is important because they may help prevent falls and fractures even when the bones are weak.

Home safety is equally important, and a few changes can help prevent falls. This is especially important for people with poor eyesight, seizures, medicines that cause dizziness, or other health conditions that may contribute to falling. Safety measures to help prevent falls include footwear, walking aids, and home modifications.[185, 186]

Walking barefoot or in socks increases the risk of falls. Shoes that are made of thin material are best, along with low heels and hard soles with treads. Wood or vinyl floors may reduce the risk of falling, but carpeted floors are more forgiving when people do fall.

Hip protector pads also help prevent fractures.[187] These are shock-absorbing pads built into briefs, panties, sweat pants, or shorts similar to hip pads that are worn by football players. These can be worn all the time or selectively during the night or when falls are more likely to occur.

Walking aids such as canes and walkers can help prevent falls, but there is also a risk of tripping over a walker or cane that has not been stored properly or used correctly. Also, walking aids can give a false sense of security. The best purpose of a walking aid is to improve mobility, but proper selection and training may help decrease the risk of falling.

Home modifications can decrease the frequency of falls.[186] In addition:

- Proper lighting at night is important. Keeping a flashlight at the bedside and using it is a simple method. Also, nightlights in the hallways and bathrooms improve visibility at night. This is especially important for pet owners to avoid tripping over the pet animal during the night.

- Remove small throw rugs. These are a potential source of trouble because they are uneven with the rest of the flooring and may shift in position.

- Keep floors and stairways clear of small objects or clothing.

- Make sure chairs, stools, and other furniture are stable with good support at the edges and corners in case someone sits on the edge of the furniture.

• If balance is a problem, then install hand rails in the bathroom and add adhesive surfaces to the floor of the tub or shower.

Medicines for Osteoporosis

Bisphosphonates taken by mouth include alendronate (Fosamax®), risedronate (Actonel®), Etidronate (Didronel®), and ibandronate (Boniva®). Zolendronate (Aclasta®) is an intravenous form of bisphosphonates, although some of the oral types can also be given intravenously.

It's recommended to take these on an empty stomach with eight ounces of water half an hour before any food, drinks, or other medicines. Sitting or standing for thirty to sixty minutes after taking bisphosphonates is also recommended to help avoid heartburn or indigestion.[188, 189]

Bisphosphonates are deposited on the surface of bones, where they slow down bone loss by decreasing the activity of osteoclasts, the cells that take away bone during the process of bone maintenance.[189] The osteoclasts then undergo apoptosis, which is another name for premature cell death. More can form, but the original ones disappear. These medicines have been used for over thirty years and are generally the first choice for treatment of osteoporosis.[12]

Bisphosphonates decrease the risk of a second fracture in women with osteoporosis who have already had a fracture. Reviews based on the best available evidence, however, concluded that the benefits are less for preventing the first fracture.[170-172] These studies reported that bisphosphonates are about the same as vitamin D and calcium for preventing fractures in women with low bone mineral density who have never had a fragility fracture.

This is partly because many women with low bone density never break a bone, so giving bisphosphonates to everyone with low bone density doesn't make a big enough difference to be detected statistically. Low bone mineral density is only one factor in determining bone strength, but it is an important factor for those who actually break their bones. For the people with weak bones that break, one way to strengthen the bone is to increase bone mineral density with bisphosphonates.

A major problem with bisphosphonates is that approximately half of the people who are treated will stop taking the medicine within a year after beginning.[190] This is a problem whether the medicine is taken once a week or once a month.[191] The most common complaints include indigestion, nausea, heartburn, or irritation of the lining of the throat or stomach.[12]

Serious complications are rare, although some can be major problems—such as osteonecrosis of the jaw, where the bone in the jaw has poor circulation. This increases the risk of serious infections, which are difficult to treat after tooth extraction. This occurs approximately once in 10,000 patients, including some otherwise healthy patients.[190, 192]

A study of this condition, however, found that nine out of ten cases of osteonecrosis of the jaw occurred following intravenous zolendronate treatment, and in patients with cancer, mainly one type of cancer called *multiple myeloma*.[193] In spite of this concern, studies show that bisphosphonate treatment decreases two-to-five year mortality rates by more than 10%, especially in older more frailer individuals.[194, 195] Some of this improved life expectancy is because of fewer hip fractures.[195]

Another complication is unusual fractures, especially stress fractures and fractures just below the hip. These are called *atypical fractures* and may develop because the bone can't repair microscopic damage that accumulates over a period of years.[195]

My mother had an atypical fracture, and these are more difficult to treat than other types of broken bones. The good news is that orthopedic surgeons are improving the methods to treat these types of fractures. Another consideration is to stop taking bisphosphonates after five years because the benefits continue for several years, and taking a break from these medicines might give the bone a chance to repair the microdamage.[195]

In summary, the greatest benefits from bisphosphonates are in women with osteoporosis who have already had one or more fractures. The benefits of bisphosphonates may also outweigh the risks for women with osteoporosis and other risk factors, but this is less clear.

Hormone Replacement Therapy (HRT) is reported to improve bone mineral density, but long-term treatment is associated with increased rates of breast cancer, heart attack, stroke, and blood clots.[188] For this reason, treatment with estrogen and progestin have generally been stopped as a treatment for osteoporosis. Short-term treatment may be useful to help manage problems during early stages of menopause, but long-term treatment with increasing age has greater risks. [196]

Selective Estrogen Receptor Modulators (SERM) is a drug that works by targeting places where estrogen binds to various types of tissues. The drug raloxifene (Evista®) is a SERM, but there are many types of SERMs. Only a few act specifically to improve bone metabolism. Other types may act to reduce the risk of breast cancer without any effect on bone. The one that is mostly used for osteoporosis is called raloxifene, although there may be more in the future.

Raloxifene has been most effective for reducing the risk of vertebral fractures, even though there is limited improvement in bone mineral density. This suggests that raloxifene may improve other properties of bone strength, in addition to the mineral content.[188] The benefits for bones other than the spine have been insignificant.[188] Another benefit of raloxifine has been a decrease in risk of breast cancer.

There is an increase, however, in the risk of stroke and dangerous blood clots for women taking raloxifene.[192, 197] The frequency of hot flashes and leg cramps may also be increased in some women taking raloxifene.

In summary, raloxifene increases the risk of blood clots in the legs, but may be useful for women with osteoporosis who also have a high risk for breast cancer.

Calcitonin, in the form of salmon calcitonin, has been available for many years. It is a hormone that decreases the activity of osteoclasts and decreases the rate of bone loss. Calcitonin slows down the bone remodeling, similar to bisphosphonates, except that calcitonin does not cause premature death of the osteoclast cells.[198] Calcitonin can be used for children, during pregnancy, and while breast feeding, and no toxic effects have been reported.[12]

One problem with calcitonin is that it must be taken by injection or by nasal spray, although oral forms are being developed. The injections may cause nausea, headaches, and flushing, while the nasal spray may cause congestion or irritation of the nasal passages. Another problem is that some studies show calcitonin is not as effective as bisphosphonates for preventing hip fractures, even though it is similar to bisphosphonates for prevention of spine fractures.[199]

In summary, calcitonin is generally used as a second choice for patients who don't tolerate bisphosphonates. It is also useful in certain types of rare bone diseases, such as children with osteoporosis, or in women who are pregnant.

Parathyroid hormone, or a synthetic form called teriparatide (Forteo®), may be given by daily injections for the treatment of osteoporosis. This hormone improves several aspects of bone strength, including bone formation and repair.[12] Supplementation with calcium and vitamin D is usually recommended to improve the effects.[12, 188] Increased bone mineral density and decreased number of fractures have been reported for people using teriparatide.[188, 197]

Problems with teriparatide include headaches, nausea, and dizziness after injection. A bigger concern, however, is possible increased risk of bone cancer.[118, 197] This has been reported in studies using experimental animals but is rare in humans taking teriparatide, with an estimated rate of one per 100,000 patients. For comparison, the risk of bone cancer in the general population is approximately one in 250,000 people. Since there is a slightly increased risk of bone cancer, teriparatide is usually recommended only for twenty-four months for severe osteoporosis.

In summary, teriparatide is usually recommended for patients who have had more fractures while taking bisphosphonates, or for patients with established osteoporosis who cannot tolerate bisphosphonates.[197]

RANKL inhibitors, also called RANK-Ligand inhibitors, include denosumab (Prolia®) that is approved for use for osteoporosis and other causes of bone loss. This is a more recent addition to the list of medicines that may be used to treat osteoporosis, so denosumab has not been studied as long as some of the other medicines. Denosumab is given by injection twice a year, and few side effects have been reported.[200]

This medicine is designed to attack a protein that tells osteoclasts to take away bone. When this protein is stopped, then the bone loss is slowed down. Denosumab slows down the osteoclasts, but it does not cause cell death like bisphosphonates. There have been reports, however, of osteonecrosis of the jaw, and there may be future problems with atypical fractures because of limited ability to remodel microscopic bone damage.[118]

Studies in humans over a period of three years have shown effective prevention of fractures similar to intravenous bisphosphonates, or synthetic parathyroid hormone.[200, 201] Denosumab is well-tolerated, but a very slightly increased risk of infections of the skin, ear, and bladder have been reported.[118] The risk of this type of infection in approximately one in 10,000 patients taking the medicine.

In summary, denosumab is a relatively recent addition to the medicines that can be used for osteoporosis. It seems to work as well as bisphosphonates and may be tolerated better, but requires injections twice a year.

Strontium ranelate was discussed earlier in this book. Currently, it is not approved for use in the United States. Studies using two grams a day have reported decreased fracture rates similar to bisphosphonates without major side effects, except for a slight increase in the risk of blood clots compared to placebo.[118] Strontium is a metal that replaces calcium, stays in the bone for a long time, and makes the bone appear more dense on X-ray tests.

Recovering from a Fracture

Anyone who breaks a bone after the age of fifty should check with his or her primary care physician to be evaluated for bone health and for conditions that may affect bone health.

Studies show that fewer than one-third of patients with a fragility fracture are evaluated for bone mineral density.[202] The American Orthopedic Association has initiated a national program to improve the frequency of evaluation after fragility fractures, but the individual can also help by asking the doctors to see if the break occurred because of weak bones.

Hip fractures. The important points in the first few weeks after a broken hip are:

1. Early surgical treatment as soon as the medical condition permits. Lying in bed is unhealthy for older people, so it's important to get the broken

bone fixed and stable without unnecessary delays. Delays longer than two days are associated with increased mortality after a hip fracture, but this measure may also mean that delays are more common in people who are sicker when they break their hip.[12]

2. Rapid mobilization after surgery. This means that sitting, standing, and walking will begin as soon as possible after surgery. This may be painful or difficult, but getting out of bed saves lives by preventing blood clots, pressure sores, pneumonia, and other complications after surgery. Stable fixation of the broken bone helps manage the pain, but brittle bones are more difficult to hold together with metal implants.

3. Return to normal activities as soon as possible. Rehabilitation will help build strength and independence. The daily routine in a home environment is good therapy after a broken hip.

Recovery after other fractures. Any broken bone after the age of fifty is a warning sign:

1. It's important to protect the broken bone while it heals, but it's also important to be as active as possible after a broken bone. Inactivity causes muscle weakness and bone loss in other parts of the skeleton. Even with a broken shoulder or wrist, it's important to continue walking or other exercises to maintain bone health.

2. Be especially careful of falling while recovering from a broken bone. Even a short period of bed rest can cause problems with balance and coordination. Also, pain medicines can cause dizziness, and balance problems that add to the risk of falling. It's best to be careful by holding onto someone, or by using handrails or a walker because of the possibility or sudden loss of balance.

3. Get tested for bone mineral density following any fragility fracture. This includes broken wrists or ankles that are often ignored after they heal. These are common signs of brittle bones that go unrecognized until

something worse happens.

4. As soon as you recover from the broken bone, it's important to improve your exercise and nutrition to make up for the ground that's been lost. After a broken bone, extra nutrition and extra exercise for a few months are needed to recover what's been lost.

It's not enough simply to return to your old level of activity. Recovery also takes two to three times longer than most people realize, so you should plan several months of extra effort for full recovery.

Tips for Getting Started on Your Bone Health Program

Nutrition: Good nutrition can begin immediately by finding wholesome foods you enjoy and substituting them for other eating habits. Change the water you're drinking and eat more dried fruits and dry roasted nuts.

Instead of ice cream for dessert, try peach yogurt with fresh blueberries. Even strawberry shortcake with plenty of strawberries and low-fat topping is healthier than cake.

Purchase organic vegetables and eat some fresh spinach salad, topped with bacon bits, boiled egg, and poppyseed dressing. Another healthy salad is spring mix lettuces with walnuts, dried cherries, and raspberry vinaigrette dressing. Also, getting enough meats and protein without going overboard is important for bone health.

Supplement your diet with the nutrients that you may be lacking, and don't go overboard with megadoses unless there's a specific reason to take a lot of one nutrient.

When possible, avoid over-the-counter medicines that may interfere with bone health. These include too much ibuprofen and naproxen. It also includes some of the medicines called *proton pump inhibitors* that are taken to decrease heartburn and indigestion. Also, too much vitamin A can reduce bone mineral density.

Medical care: Get a regular check-up with your doctor. Ask him or her if you need a bone mineral density test. An examination and blood tests can detect other problems before they develop, and you can make sure you're healthy enough to begin a more rigorous exercise program.

Exercise: How can you find time to exercise when you already have a busy schedule and too many activities to get done each day? Approximately nineteen out of twenty adults exercise less than 30 minutes a day and less than two and a half hours a week.[203] If you are one of those nineteen who don't exercise enough, you need to change your habits. You'll feel better, live longer, and be healthier if you have some modest exercise regularly.

- Choose an activity that appeals to you. This might be dancing, walking, dusting off the tennis racquet, playing golf (walking, not riding in a cart), volleyball, basketball, or weight lifting. Even swimming is healthy, although it's not quite as good for bones as impact activities like tennis and jogging.
- Find a friend if you can. On days you don't want to exercise, your buddy will drag you out—and you'll do the same for him or her.
- Either set aside five days a week for half an hour, or set aside two days a week for an hour or more of exercise. You can find the time and make a commitment.

Pick one habit at a time to fix. Don't expect success if you suddenly decide to exercise, diet, stop smoking, watch less television, and sleep more all at the same time.

- Make a thirty-day commitment. Focus on thirty days and don't think about a lifetime commitment. You can re-evaluate after the first thirty days. At least you'll be healthier if you decide to change things after the first effort. If you've found the right schedule and activity, then you can continue and begin to work on the next improvement

- Choose a short, simple ritual that gets you into the activity. This can help condition you to begin. It may be as simple as setting an alarm clock or a fifteen-minute warning on your iPhone. It could be drinking a glass of water, putting on a wristband, or almost anything simple that says, "We're starting *now.*"

- Write it down. Make a calendar or list with the times and dates you'll exercise. Then check them off for the first thirty days. This will give you a sense of commitment and also a sense of accomplishment when you check off the days.

- Be patient, and don't expect to feel different or look different right away. It may be several months before others begin to notice the change in your health.

.

REFERENCES

1.   Price, C, Connolly JF, Carantzas AC, Ilyas I, *Comparison of bone grafts for posterior spinal fusion in adolescent idiopathic scoliosis.* Spine, 2003. **28**(8): p. 793-8.

2.   Knapp, DR, Jones ET, Blanco JS, Flynn JC, Price CT, *Allograft bone in spinal fusion for adolescent idiopathic scoliosis.* J. Spinal Disorders and Techniques, 2005. **18S**: p. S73-6.

3.   Hing, K, Wilson LF, Buckland T, *Comparative performance of three ceramic bone graft substututes.* Spine J, 2007. **7**(4): p. 475-90.

4.   Coathup, M, Samizadeh S, Fang YS, Buckland T, Hing, KA, Blunn GW, *The osteoinductivity of silicate-substututed calcium phosphate.* J. Bone and Joint Surg, 2011. **93A**(23): p. 2219-6.

5.   Välimäki, V-V, Aro HT, *Molecular basis for action of bioactive glasses as bone graft substututes.* Scand. J. Surg., 2006. **95**: p. 95-102.

6.   Waked, W, Grauer J, *Silicates and bone fusion.* Orthopedics, 2008. **31**(6): p. 591-7.

7.   Piotrowski, G, Hench LL, Allen WC, Miller GJ, *Mechanical studies of the bone bioglass interfacial bond.* J. Biomed. Mater Res, 1975. **9**(4): p. 47-61.

8.   Melton, L, Kan SH, Wahner HW, Riggs BL, *Lifetime fracture risk: an approach to hip fracture risk assessment based on bone mineral density and age.* J. Clin. Epidemiol, 1988. **41**(10): p. 985-94.

9.   Einhorn, T, *Metabolic Bone Disease*, in *Orthopaedic Basic Science*, T.A. Einhorn, O'Keefe RJ, Buckwalter JA, Editor. 2007, American Academy of Orthopedic Surgeons: Rosemont. p. 4125-26.

10. United States Department of Health and Human Services, *Bone Health and Osteoporosis: a report of the Surgeon General*, 2004, Office of the Surgeon General: Rockville, MD.

11. Orwoll, E, Vanek C, *Atlas of Osteoporosis*. 3rd ed, editor E.S. Orwoll. 2009, Philadelphia: Springer.

12. Bartl, R., Frisch B, *Osteoporosis: Diagnosis, Prevention, Treatment*. Second ed. 2004, Heidelberg: Springer-Verlag.

13. Noris-Suarez, K, Lira-Olivares J, Ferrira AM, Feijoo JL, Suarez N, Hernandez MC, Barrios E, *In vitro deposition of hydroxyapatite on cortical bone collagen stimulated by deformation-induced piezoelectricity*. Biomacromolecules, 2007. **8**(3): p. 941-8.

14. Nomura, S, Takano-Yamamoto T, *Molecular events caused by mechanical stress in bone*. Matrix Biol, 2000. **19**(2): p. 91-6.

15. Miclau, T, Bozic KJ, Tay B, et.al., *Bone injury, regeneration, and repair*, in *Orthopedic Basic Science: Foundations of Clinical Practice*, T.A. Einhorn, O'Keefe RJ, Buckwalter JA, Editor. 2007, American Adacemy of Orthopedic Surgeons: Rosemont. p. 331-48.

16. Carlisle, E.M., *Silicon: a possible factor in bone calcification*. Science, 1970. **167**: p. 179-80.

17. Mineral Information Institute (Lead Author);Sidney Draggan (Topic Editor) "*Silicon*". In: Encyclopedia of Earth. Eds. Cutler J. Cleveland (Washington, D.C.: Environmental Information Coalition, National Council for Science and the Environment). [First published in the Encyclopedia of Earth January 17, 2008; Last revised Date March 1, 2011; Retrieved February 14, *2012 http://www.eoearth.org/article/Silicon*

18. Martin, K, *The chemistry of silica and its potential health benefits*. J. Nutrition, Health and Aging, 2007. **11**(2): p. 94-98.

19. United States Food and Drug Administration, *FDA update on the safety of silicone gel-filled breast implants*, Center for Devices and Radiological Health, Editor. 2011: Washington, D.C.

20. Takizawa, Y, Hirasawa F, Noritomo E, Aida M, Tsunoda H, Uesugi S, *Oral ingestion of syloid to mice and rats and its chronic toxicity and carcinogenicity*. Acta. Medica et Biologica, 1988. **36**: p. 27-56.

21. Aguilar, F, Charrondiere UR, Dusemund B, et.al., *Scientific Opinion: Monomethylsilanetriol added for nutritional purposes to food supplements*. European Food Safety Authority Journal, 2009. **950**: p. 1-12.

22. National Academy of Sciences, *Dietary reference intakes for vitamin A, vitamin K, arsenic, boron, chromium, copper, iodine, iron, manganese, molybdenum, nickel, silicon, vanadium, and zinc*, National Institutes of Health (NIH), Editor. 2001, National Academies Press: Washington.

23. Jugdaohsingh, R, *Silicon and bone health*. J. Nutrition, Health and Aging, 2007. **11**: p. 99-110.

24. Schwarz, K, Milne DB, *Growth promoting effects of silicon in rats*. Nature, 1972. **239**: p. 333-4.

25. Gitelman, H, Alderman FR, Perry SJ, *Silicon accumulation in dialysis patients*. Am. J. Kidney Dis., 1992. **19**(2): p. 140-3.

26. Munger, R, Cerhan JR, Bhiu BC-H, *Prospective study of dietary protein intake and risk of hip fracture in post-menopausal women*. Am J Clin Nutr, 1999. **69**: p. 147-52.

27. Hott, M, de Pollak C, Modrowski D, Marie PJ, *Short-term effects of organic silicon on trabecular bone in mature ovariectomized rats*. Calcif. Tissue Int., 1993. **53**: p. 174-9.

28. Seaborn, C, Nielsen FH, *Dietary silicon affects acid and alkaline phosphatase and $^{45}Calcium$ uptake in bone of rats*. J. Trace Elements Exp. Med., 1994. **7**: p. 11-18.

29. Seaborn, C, Nielsen FH, *Dietary silicon and arginine affect mineral element composition of rat femur and vertebra*. Biol. Trace Elem. Res., 2002. **89**: p. 239-50.

30. Küçükbay, F, Yazlak H, Sahin N, Akdemir F, Orhan C, Juturu V, Sahin K, *Effects of dietary arginine silicate inositol complex on mineral status in rainbow trout (Oncorhynchus mykiss)*. Aquaculture Nutr., 2008. **14**(3): p. 257-62.

31. Nielsen, B, Potter GD, Morris EL, et.al., *Training distance to failure in young racing quarter horses fed sodium zeolite A*. J. Equine Vet. Sci., 1993. **13**(10): p. 562-7.

32. Rico, H, Gallego-Lago JL, Hernandez ER, Villa LF, Sanchez-Atrio A, Seco C, Gervas JJ, *Effect of silicon supplement on osteopenia induced by ovariectomy in rats*. Calcif. Tissue Int., 2000. **66**: p. 53-5.

33. Bae, Y, Kim JY, Choi MK, Chung YS, Kim MH, *Short-term administration of water-soluble silicon improves mineral denstiy of femur and tibia in ovariectomized rats*. Biol. Trace Elem. Res., 2008. **124**: p. 157-63.

34. Calomme, M, Geusens P, Demeester N, Behets GJ, D'Haese P, Sindambiwe JB, Vanden Berghe D, *Partial prevention of long-term femoral bone loss in aged ovariectomized rats supplemented with choline-stabilized orthosilicic acid.* Calcif. Tissue Int., 2006. **78**(4): p. 227-32.

35. Kim, M, Bae YJ, Choi MK, Chung YS, *Silicon supplementation improves the bone mineral density of calcium-deficient ovariectomized rats by reducing bone resorption.* Biol. Trace Elem. Res., 2009. **128**: p. 239-47.

36. Jugdaosingh, R, Tucker KL, Qiao N, Cupples LA, Kiel DP, Powell JJ, *Dietary silicon intake is positively associated with bone mineral density in men and premenopausal women of the Framingham offspring cohort.* J. Bone Min. Res., 2004. **19**(2): p. 297-307.

37. Macdonald, H, Hardcastle AE, Jugdaosingh R, Reid DM, *Dietary silicon intake is associated with bone mineral density in premenopausal women and postmenopausal women taking HRT.* J. Bone Min. Res., 2005. **20**: p. S393.

38. Merkley, J, Miller ER, *The effect of sodium fluoride and sodium silicate on growth and bone strength of broilers.* Poultry Sci, 1983. **62**: p. 798-804.

39. Carlisle, EM, *Silicon: a requirement in bone formation independend of Vitamin D₁.* Calcif. Tissue Int., 1981. **33**: p. 27-34.

40. McNaughton, S, Bolton-Smith C, Mishra GD, Jugdaosingh R, Powell JJ, *Dietary silicon intake in post-menopausal women.* Brit. J. Nutrition, 2005. **94**: p. 813-7.

41. Chen, F, Cole P, Wen L, Mi Z, Trapico EJ, *Estimates of trace element intakes in Chinese farmers.* J. Nutr., 1994. **124**: p. 196-201.

42. Anasuya, A, Narasinga RBS, *Effect of fluoride, silicon, and magnesium on the mineralizing capacity of an inorganic medium and stone formers urine tested by a modified in vitro method.* Biochem. Med., 1983. **30**(2): p. 146-56.

43. Johnell, O, Kanis JA, *An estimate of the worldwide prevalence, mortality and disability associated with hip fracture.* Osteoporosis Int, 2004. **15**: p. 897-902.

44. Eisinger, J, Clairet D, *Effects of silicon, fluoride, etidonate and magnesium on bone mineral density: a retrospective study.* Magnesium Res., 1993. **6**: p. 247-9.

45. Schiano, A, Eisinger F, Detolle P, Laponche AM, Brisou B, Eisinger J, *Silicium, tissu osseus et immunité.* Revue du Rhumatisme, 1979. **46**(7-9): p. 483-6.

46.   Spector, T, Calomme MR, Anderson SH, et.al., *Choline stabilized orthosilicic acit dupplementation as an adjunct to Calcium/Vitamin D3 stimulates markers of bone formation in osteopenic females: a randomized, placebo-controlled trial.* BMC Musculoskel. Disorders, 2008. **9**: p. 85-94.

47.   Li Z, Karp H, Zerlin A, Lee TY, Carpenter C, Heber D, *Absorption of silicon from artesian aquifer water and its impact on bone health in postmenopausal women: a 12 week pilot study.* Nutrition J., 2010. **9**(1): p. 44.

48.   Jugdaosingh, R, Anderson SHC, Tucker KL, Elliott H, Kiel DP, Thompson RPH, Powell JJ, *Dietary silicon intake and absorption.* Am J Clin Nutr, 2002. **75**: p. 887-93.

49.   Gilette-Guyonnet, S, Andrieu S, Vellas B, *The potential influence of silica present in drinking water on Alzheimer's disease and associated disorders.* J. Nutr., 2007. **11**(2): p. 119-24.

50.   Rabon, HJ, Roland DA Sr, Bryant MM, Smith RC, Barnes DG, Laurent SM, *Absorption of silicon and aluminum by hens fed sodium zeolite A with various levels of cholecalciferol.* Poultry Sci, 1995. **74**(2): p. 352-9.

51.   Onderci, M, Sahin N, Sahin K, Balci TA, Gursu MF, Juturu V, Kucuk O, *Dietary arginine silicate inositol complex during the late laying period of quail at different environmental temperatures.* Br. Poult Sci, 2006. **47**(2): p. 209-15.

52.   Sahin, K, Onderci M, Sahin T, Balci TA, Gursu MF, Juturu V, Kucuk O, *Dietary arginine silicate inositol complex improves bone mineralization in quail.* Poultry Sci, 2006. **85**: p. 486-92.

53.   Price, CT, editor, *Instructional Course Lectures: Volume 49*, 2000, Rosemont, Illinois: American Academy of Orthopedic Surgeons.

54.   Celotti, F, Bignamini A, *Dietary calcium and mineral/vitamin supplementation: a controversial problem.* J. Intl. Medical Res., 1999. **27**(1): p. 1-14.

55.   Bolland, M, Grey A, Avenell A, Gambel GD, Reid IR, *Calcium supplements with or without vitamin D and risk of cardiovascular events: reanalysis of Women's Health Initiative limited access dataset and meta-analysis.* Br. Med. J, 2011. **342**(April 19): p. d2040.

56.   Bischoff-Ferrari, H, Dawson-Hughes B, Baron JA, et.al., *Calcium intake and hip fracture risk in men and women: a meta-analysis of prospective cohort studies and randomized controlled trials.* Am J Clin Nutr, 2007. **86**: p. 1780-90.

57. Guéguen, L, Pointillart A, *The bioavailability of dietary calcium.* J. Am Coll Nutr, 2000. **19**(2): p. 119S-136S.

58. National Institutes of Health (NIH), *Calcium: dietary supplement fact sheet,* in *Office of Dietary Supplements,* NIH, Editor. 2011, U.S.

59. Bolscher, M, Netelenbos JC, Barto R, et.al., *Estrogen regulation of intestinal calcium absorption in the intact and ovariectomized adult rat.* J. Bone Min. Res., 1999. **14**(7): p. 1197-1202.

60. Volpe, S, Taper LJ, Meacham S, *The relationship between boron and magnesium status and bone mineral density in the human: a review.* Magnesium Res., 1993. **6**(3): p. 291-6.

61. Nielsen, F, Hunt CD, Mullen LM, Hunt JR, *Effect of dietary boron on mineral, estrogen, and testosterone metabolism in postmenopausal women.* FAESB J (Federation of American Societies of Experimental Biology), 1987. **1**(5): p. 394-7.

62. Bouillon, R, *Why modest but widespread improvement of the vitamin D status is the best strategy?* Best Pract Clin Endocrinol Metab, 2011. **25**(4): p. 693-62.

63. National Insitutes of Health (NIH), *Magnesium: dietary supplement fact sheet.* Office of Dietary Supplements, 2011. NIH.

64. Launius, B, Brown PA, Cush EM, Mancini MC, *Osteoporosis: the dynamic relationship between magnesium and bone mineral density in heart transplant patients.* Crit Care Nurs Q, 2004. **27**(1): p. 96-100.

65. Vormann, J, *Magnesium: nutrition and metabolism.* Molecular Aspects of Medicine, 2003. **24**(1-3): p. 27-37.

66. Rude, R, Singer FR, Gruber HE, *Skeletal and hormonal effects of magnesium deficiency.* J. Am. Coll. Nutr, 2009. **28**(2): p. 131-41.

67. Tucker, K, Hannan MT, Chen H, Cupples LA, Wilson PWF, Kiel DP, *Potassium, magnesium and fruit and vegetable intakes are associated with greater bone mineral density in elderly men and women.* Am J Clin Nutr, 1999. **69**: p. 727-36.

68. Rude, R, Gruber HE, *Magnesium deficiency and osteoporosis: animal and human observations.* J. Nutr Biochem, 2004. **15**(4): p. 710-6.

69. Stendig-Lindberg, G, Tepper R, Leichter I, *Trabecular bone density in a two year controlled trial of peroral magnesium in osteoporosis.* Magnes Res, 1993. **6**(2): p. 155-63.

70. Schaafsma, A, deVries PJF, Saris WHM, *Delay of natural bone loss by higher intakes of specific minerals and vitamins.* Crit. Rev. Food Sci. and Nutr., 2001. **41**(3): p. 225-49.

71.   Eaton, S, Eaton SB III, *Paleolithic vs modern diets: selected pathophysiological implications.* . Eur J Nutr, 2000. **39**: p. 67-70.

72.   Newnham, R, *Essentiality of boron for healthy bones and joints.* Environ. Health Perspectives, 1994. **102S**(S7): p. 83-95S.

73.   Nielsen, F, *Studies on the relationship between boron and magnesium which possibly affects the formation and maintenance of bones.* Magnesium and Trace Elem. Res, 1990. **9**(2): p. 61-9.

74.   Nielsen, F, *Facts and fallacies about boron.* Nutrition Today, 1992. **27**(3): p. 8-12.

75.   Armstrong, T, Spears JW, Crenshaw TD, Nielsen FH, *Boron supplementation of a semipurified diet for weanling pigs improves feed efficiency and bone strength characteristics and alters plasma lipid metabolites.* J. Nutr., 2000. **130**(10): p. 2575-81.

76.   Hooshmand, S, Arjmandi BH, *Viewpoint: Dried plum, an emerging functional food that may effectively improve bone health.* Ageing Res Rev, 2009. **8**: p. 122-7.

77.   Stacewicz Sapuntzakis, M, Bowen PE, Hussain EA, Damayanti-Wood BI, Farnsworth NR, *Chemical composition and potential health effects of prunes: a functional food?* Crit. Rev. Food Sci. and Nutr., 2001. **41**(4): p. 251-86.

78.   Hooshmand, S, Chai SC, Saadat RL, Payton ME, Brummel-Smith K, Arjmandi BH, *Comparative effects of dried plum and dried apple on bone in postmenopausal women.* Brit. J. Nutrition, 2011. **106**: p. 923-30.

79.   Bügel, S, *Vitamin K and bone health in adult humans,* in *Vitamins and Hormones: Vitamin K*, G. LItwack, Editor. 2008, Elsevier: Amsterdam. p. 393-416.

80.   Feskanich, D, Weber P, Willett WC, Rockett H, Booth SL, Colditz GA, *Vitamin K intake and hip fractures in women: a prospective study.* Am J Clin Nutr, 1999. **69**: p. 74-9.

81.   Shea, M, Booth SL, *Update on the role of vitamin K in skeletal health.* Nutr. Rev., 2008. **66**(10): p. 549-57.

82.   Iwamoto, J, Takeda T, Sato Y, *Menatetrenone (Vitamin K2) and bone quality in the treatment of postmenopausal osteoporosis.* Nutr. Rev., 2006. **64**(12): p. 509-17.

83.   Ushiroyama, T, Ikeda A, Ueki M, *Effect of continuous therapy with vitamin K(2) and vitamin D(3) on bone mineral density and coagulofibrinolysis function in postmenopausal women.* Maturitas, 2002. **41**(3): p. 211-21.

84. Booth, S, Tucker TL, Chen H, Hannan MT, Gagnon DR, et.al., *Dietary vitamin K intakes are associated with hip fracture but not with bone mineral density in elderly men and women.* Am J Clin Nutr, 2000. **71**(5): p. 1201-8.

85. McBean, L, Speckmann, EW, *A recognition of the interrelationships of calcium with various dietary components.* Am J Clin Nutr, 1974. **27**(6): p. 603-9.

86. Scholz-Ahrens, K, Schrezenmeir J, *Effects of bioactive substances in milk on mineral and trace element metabolism with special reference to casein phosphopeptides.* Br. J. Nutrition, 2000. **84**(S1): p. S147-S153.

87. Kayongo-Male, H, Julson JL, *Effects of high levels of dietary silocon on bone development of growing rats and turkeys fed semi-purified diets.* Biol. Trace Elem. Res., 2008. **123**: p. 191-201.

88. Abrams, S, Atkinson SA, *Calcium, magnesium, phosphorous and vitamin D fortification of complementary foods.* Am Soc Nutr Sci, 2003. **133**: p. 2994S-2999S.

89. Melhus, H, Michaelsson K, Kindmark A, Bergstrom R, Holmberg L, Malmin H, Wolk A, Ljunghall S, *Excessive dietary intake of vitamin A is associated with reduced bone mineral density and increased risk of hip fracture.* Ann Int Med, 1998. **129**: p. 770-8.

90. Penniston, K, Tanumihardjo SA, *The acute and chronic toxic effects of vitamin A.* Am J Clin Nutr, 2006. **83**(2): p. 191-201.

91. Powers, K, Smith-Weller T, Franklin GM, Longstreth WT, Swanson PD, Checkoway, *Parkinson's disease risks associated with dietary iron, manganese and other nutrient intakes.* Neurology, 2003. **60**: p. 1761-6.

92. Desai, V, Kaler SG, *Role of copper in human neurological disorders.* Am J Clin Nutr, 2008. **88**((suppl)): p. 855S-858S.

93. Wang, S, *A new target in fighting brain disease: metals,* in *The Wall Street Journal.* 2012, Dow Jones & Company: New York.

94. Bush, A, *The metallobiology of Alzheimer's disease.* Trends Neurosci, 2003. **26**(4): p. 207-14.

95. Heany, R, *The vitamin D requirement in health and disease.* J. Steroid Biochem Molec Biol, 2005. **97**: p. 13-9.

96. Holick, M, Binkley NC, Bischoff-Ferrari HA, Gordon CM, Hanley DA, Heaney RP, Murad MH, Weaver CM, *Evaluation, treatment, and prevention of vitamin D deficiency: an endocrine society clinical practice guideline.* J Clin Endocrinol Metab, 2011. **96**(7): p. 1911-30.

97.   National Health and Medical Research Council, *Nutrient Reference Values for Australia and New Zealand*, Department of Health and Ageing, Editor. 2005, Australian Government, Ministry of Health.

98.   European-Food-Safety-Authority, *"Tolerable upper intake levels for vitamins and minerals"*, Scientific Committee on Food. *http://www.efsa.europa.eu/en/ndatopics/docs/ndatolerableuil.pdf.* 2006.

99.   Holden, J, Wolf WR, Mertz W, *Zinc and copper in self-selected diets.* J Am Diet Assoc, 1979. **75**(23-38).

100.   Patterson, K, Holbrook JT, Bodner JE, Kelsay JL, Smith JC Jr, Veillon C, *Zinc, copper, and manganese intake and balance for adults consuming self-selected diets.* Am J Clin Nutr, 1984. **40**(6 Suppl): p. 1397-403.

101.   National Institutes of Health (NIH) (2011) *Zinc: Dietary Supplement Fact Sheet.* Office of Dietary Supplements.

102.   Ervin, R, Wang CY, Wright JD, Kennedy-Stephens J, *Dietary intake of selected minerals for the United States population: 1999-2000.* Advanced data from vital health statistics, 2004. **no. 341**(Hyattsville, MD: National Center for Health Statistics).

103.   Fulgoni, VI, Keast DR, Bailey RL, Dwyer J, *Foods, forticants, and supplements: where do Americans get their nutrients?* J Nutr, 2011. **141**: p. 1847-54.

104.   Vinas, B, Garga LR, Ngo J, Gurinovic M, et.al., *Projected prevalence of inadequate nutrient intakes in Europe.* Ann Nutr Metab, 2011. **59**: p. 84-95.

105.   Andriollo-Sanchez, M, Hininger-Favier I, Meunier N, Toti E, et.al., *Zinc intake and status in middle-aged and older European subjects: the ZENITH study.* Eur J Clin Nutr, 2005. **59**(Suppl 2): p. S37-S41.

106.   Scientific Committee on Food, *Opinion of the Scientific Committee on Food on the Tolerable Upper Intake Level of Zinc*,Health and Consumer Protection
        Directorate-General, Editor. 2003, European Commission: Brussels.

107.   Maret, W, Sandstead HH, *Zinc requirements and the risks and benefits of zinc supplementation.* J. Trace Elements in Medicine and Biology, 2006. **20**: p. 3-18.

108.   Mursu, J, Robien K, Harnack LJ, Park K, Jacobs, Jr DR, *Dietary supplements and mortality rate in older women.* Arch Intern Med, 2011. **171**(18): p. 1625-33.

109.   Nielsen, S, *The biological role of strontium.* Bone, 2004. **35**: p. 583-8.

110. Meunier, P, Roux C, Seeman E, Ortolani S, et.al., *The effects of strontium ranelate on the risk of vertebral fracture in women with postmenopausal osteoporosis.* NEJM, 2004. **350**: p. 459-68.

111. Deeks, E, Dhillon S, *Strontium Ranelate: a review of its use in the treatment of postmenopausal osteoporosis.* Drugs, 2010. **70**(6): p. 733-59.

112. Rubin, M, Bilezikian JP, *New anabolic therapies in osteoporosis.* Rheum., 2002. **14**: p. 433-40.

113. Reginster, J-Y, Kaufman J-M, Geomaere S, Devogalaer JP, et.al., *Maintenance of antifracture efficacy over 10 years with strontium ranelate in postmenopausal osteoporosis.* Osteoporosis Int, 2012. **23**: p. 1115-22.

114. Zefirov, A, Grigor'ev PN, *Sensitivity of intracellular calcium-binding sites for exo- and endocytosis of synaptic vesicles to Sr, Ba, and Mg ions.* Neurosci Behav Physiol, 2010. **40**(4): p. 389-96.

115. Bukharaeva, E, Samigullin D, Nikolsky EE, Magazanik LG, *Modulation of kinetics of evoked quantal release at mouse neuromuscular junctions by calcium and strontium.* J. Neurochem, 2007. **100**(4): p. 939-49.

116. Cordeiro, J, Gonçalves PP, Dunant Y, *Synaptic vesicles control the time course of neurotransmitter secretion via the Ca^{2+}/H^+ antiport.* J. Physiol, 2011. **589**(1): p. 149-67.

117. Bartley, J, Reber EF, *Toxic effects of stable strontium in young pigs.* J Nutr, 1961. **75**: p. 21-8.

118. Rizzoli, R, Reginster J-Y, Boonen S, Bréart G, et.al. , *Adverse reactions and drug-drug interactions in the management of women with postmenopausal osteoporosis.* Calcif. Tissue Int., 2011. **89**: p. 91-104.

119. Blake, G, Fogelman I, *Long-term effect of strontium ranelate treatment on BMD.* J. Bone and Min. Res., 2005. **20**(11): p. 1901-4.

120. Mear, F, Yot P, Cambon M, Ribes M, *The characterization of waste cathode-ray tube glass.* Waste Manag, 2006. **26**(12): p. 1468-76.

121. Ozgür, S, Sümer H, Koço lu G, *Rickets and soil strontium.* Arch Dis Child, 1996. **75**(6): p. 524-6.

122. Sowden, E, *Trace elements in human tissue.* Biochem J, 1958. **70**(4): p. 712-5.

123. Public Health Agency for Toxic Substances and Disease Registry, *Toxicological profile for strontium*, United States Department of Health and Human Services, Editor. 2004, http://www.atsdr.cdc.gov/ToxProfiles/TP.asp?id=656&tid=120: Washington.

124. Udowenko, M, Trojan T, *Vitamin D: extent of deficiency, effect on muscle function, bone health, performance, and injury prevention.* Conn. Med. , 2010. **74**(8): p. 477-80.

125. Latham, N, Anderson CS, Reid IR, *Effects of vitamin D supplementation on strength, physical performance, and falls in older persons: a systematic review.* J Am Geriatr Soc, 2003. **51**: p. 1219-26.

126. Ceglia, L, *Vitamin D and its role in skeletal muscle.* Curr Opin Clin Nutr Metab Care, 2009(12): p. 628-33.

127. Autier, P, Gandini S, *Vitamin D supplementation and total mortality.* Arch Intern Med, 2007. **167**(16): p. 1730-7.

128. Gartner, ., Greer FR, *Prevention of rickets and vitamin D deficiency: new guidelines for vitamin D intake.* Pediatrics, 2003. **111**: p. 908-10.

129. Glowacki, J, Hurwitz S, Thornhill TS, Kelly M, LeBoff MS, *Osteoporosis and vitamin-D deficiency among postmenopausal women with osteoarthritis undergoing total hip arthroplasty.* J. Bone and Joint Surg, 2003. **85A**(12): p. 2371-7.

130. Rosen, C, *Vitamin D insufficiency.* NEJM, 2011. **364**: p. 248-54.

131. Bischoff-Ferrari, H, Willett WC, Wong JB, Giovannucci E, Dietrich T, Dawson-Hughes B, *Fracture prevention with vitamin D supplementation: a meta-analysis of randomized controlled trials.* JAMA, 2005. **293**: p. 2257-64.

132. Sahni, S, Hannan MT, Gagnon D, Blumberg J, Cupples LA, Kiel DP, Tucker KL, *Protective effect of total and supplemental vitamin C intake on the risk of hip fracture —a 17 year follow-up from the Framingham Osteoporosis Study.* Osteoporosis Int, 2009. **20**(11): p. 1853-61.

133. Chuin, A, Labonte M, Tessier D, Khalil A, Bobeuf F, Doyon CY, Reigh N, Dionne IJ, *Effect of antioxidants combined to resistance training on BMD in elderly women: a pilot study* Osteoporosis Int, 2009. **20**(7): p. 1253-8.

134. Leveille, S, LaCroix AZ, Koepsell TD, et.al., *Dietary vitamin C and bone mineral density in postmenopausal women in Washington State, USA.* J. Epidem and Commun Health, 1997. **51**(5): p. 479-85.

135. Grases, F, Sanchis P, Prieto RM, Perello J, Lopez-Gonzalez AA, *Effect of tetracalcium dimagnesium phytate on bone characteristics in ovaiectomized rats.* J Medicinal Foods, 2010. **13**(6): p. 1301-6.

136. Thomas, W, Tilden MT, *Inhibition of mineralization by hydrolysates of phytic acid.* Hopkins Med J, 1972. **131**: p. 133-42.

137. López-González, A, Grases F, Roca P, et.al., *Phytate (myo-Inositol Hexaphosphate) and risk factors for osteoporosis.* J. Medicinal Foods, 2008. **11**(4): p. 747-52.

138. Dai, Z, Chung SK, Miao D, Lau KS, Chan AW, Kung AW, *Sodium/myo-inositol cotransporter 1 and myo-inositol are essential for osteogenesis and bone formation.* J. Bone Min. Res., 2011. **26**(3): p. 582-90.

139. Angeloff, L, Skoryna SC, Henderson IWD, *Effects of the hexahydroxyhexane myoinositol on bone uptake of radiocalcium in rats: Effect of inositol and vitamin D_2 on bone uptake of ^{45}Ca in rats.* Acta Pharmacol Toxicol (Copenh), 1977. **40**(2): p. 209-15.

140. Falsafi, R, Tatakis DN, Hagel-Bradway S, Dziak R, *Effects of inositol trisphosphate on calcium mobilization in bone cells.* Calcif. Tissue Int., 1991. **49**: p. 333-9.

141. Tong, B, Barbul A, *Cellular and physiological effects of arginine.* Mini Rev Med Chem, 2004. **4**(8): p. 823-32.

142. Corbett, S, McCarthy ID, Batten J, Hukkanen M, Polak JM, Hughes SPF, *Nitric oxide mediated vasoreactivity during fracture repair.* Clin Orthop Rel Res, 1999. **365**: p. 247-53.

143. McCarty, M, *Supplemental arginine and high-dose folate may promote bone health by supporting the activity of endothelial-type nitric oxide synthase in bone.* Med Hypotheses, 2005. **64**(5): p. 1030-3.

144. Kdolsky, R, Reihsner R, Beer R, *Biomechanical analysis of fracture healing in guinea-pigs.* Studies in Health Technol. and Informatics, 2008. **133**: p. 141-7.

145. Dirschl, D, Henderson RC, Oakley WC, *Accelerated bone mineral loss following a hip fracture: a prospective longitudinal follow-up.* Bone, 1997. **21**(1): p. 79-82.

146. Powell JJ, McNaughton SA, Jugdaosingh R, Anderson SHC, Dear J, Knot F, et.al., *A provisional database for the silicon content of foods in the United Kingdom.* Brit. J. Nutrition, 2005. **94**: p. 804-12.

147. Bellia, J, Birchall JD, Roberts NB, *Beer: a dietary sourde of silicon.* Lancet, 1994. **343**: p. 235.

148. Pedrera-Zamoano, J, Lavado-Garcia JM, Roncero-Martin R, Calderon-Garcia JF, et.al., *Effect of beer drinking on ultrasound bone mass in women.* Nutrition, 2009. **25**(10): p. 1057-63.

149. Tucker, K, Jugdaosingh R, Powell JJ, et.al., *Effects of beer, wine, and liquor intakes on bone mineral density in older men and women.* Am J Clin Nutr, 2009. **89**: p. 1188-96.

150. Sripanyakorn, S, Jugdaosingh R, Dissayabutr W, Anderson SHC, Thompson RPH, Powell JJ *The comparative absorption of silicon from different foods and food supplements.* Brit. J. Nutrition, 2009. **102**: p. 825-34.

151. Giammarioli, S, Mosca M, Sanzini E, *Silicon content of Italian mineral waters and its contribution to daily intake.* J Food Sci, 2005. **70**: p. S509-S512.

152. Chan, K, Anderson M, Lau EMC, *Exercise interventions: defusing the world's osteoporosis time bomb.* Bull. World Health Org, 2003. **81**(11): p. 827-30.

153. Faucett, S, Genuario JW, Tosteson ANA, Koval KJ, *Is prophylactic fixation a cost-efficient method to prevent a future contralateral fragility hip fracture?* J. Orthop. Trauma, 2010. 24(2): p. 65-74

154. Haleem, S, Lutchman L, Mayahi, R, *Mortality following hip fracture: trends and geographical variations over the last 40 years.* Injury, Int. J. Care Injured, 2008. **39**: p. 1157-63.

155. Koh, L, Sedrine WB, Torralba TB, Kung A, et.al., *A simple tool to identify Asian women at increased risk of osteoporosis.* Osteoporosis Int, 2001. **12**: p. 699-705.

156. Geusens, P, Hochberg MC, van der Voort DJ, Pols H, van der Klift M, Siris E, Melton Me, Turpin J, Byrnes C, Ross P, *Performance of risk indices for identifying low bone density in postmenopausal women.* Mayo Clin Proc, 2002. **77**: p. 629-37.

157. Rud, B, Jensen JEB, Mosekilde L, Nielsen SP, Hilden J, Abrahamsen B, *Performance of four clinical screening tools to select peri- and early postmenopausal women for dual x-ray absorptiometry.* Osteoporosis Int, 2005. **16**: p. 764-72.

158. Skedros, J, Sybrowsky CL, Stoddard GJ, *The Osteoporosis Self-assessment Screening Tool: a useful tool for the orthopaedic surgeon.* J. Bone and Joint Surg, 2007. **89A**(4): p. 765-72.

159.   Vuolteenaho, K, Moilanen T, Moilanen E, *Non-steroidal anti-inflammatory drugs, cyclooxygenase-2 and the bone healing process.* Basic Clin Pharmacol Toxicol, 2008. **102**(1): p. 10-4.

160.   Eom, C, Park SM, Myung SK, Yun JM, Ahn JS, *Use of acid-suppressive drugs and risk of fracture: a meta-analysis of observational studies.* Am Fam Med, 2011. **9**(3): p. 257-67.

161.   National Institutes of Health (NIH), *Vitamin A and Carotenoids: Dietary Supplement Fact Sheet.* . Office of Dietary Supplements, 2011.

162.   Kanis, J, Johnell O, Oden A, et.al. , *FRAX® and the assessment of fracture probability in nem and women from the UK.* Osteoporosis Int, 2008. **19**: p. 385-97.

163.   Hans, D, Kanis JA, B aim S, B ielzikian JP, Binkley N, et.al., *Joint official position of the International Society for Clinical Densitometry and International Osteoporosis Foundation on FRAX®* J clin Densitom, 2011. **14**(3): p. 240-62.

164.   Unnanuntana, A, Gladnick BP, Donnelly E, Lane JM, *The assessment of fracture risk.* J. Bone and Joint Surg, 2010. **92A**: p. 743-53.

165.   Black, DM, Steinbuch M, Palermo L, Dargent-Molina P, Lindsay R, Hoseyni MS, Johnell O, *An assessment tool for predicting fracture risk in postmenopausal women.* Osteoporosis Int, 2001. **12**: p. 519-28.

166.   Faulkner, K, Wacker WK, Barden HS, Simonelli C, Burke PK, Ragi S, Del Rio L, *Femur strength index predicts hip fracture independent of bone density and hip axis length.* Osteoporosis Int, 2006. **17**(4): p. 593-9.

167.   Kanis, J, *Diagnosis of osteoporosis and assessment of fracture risk.* Lancet, 2002. **359**: p. 1929-36.

168.   Moayyeri, A, Adams JE, Adler RA, Krieg M-A, Hans D, Compston J, Lewiecki EM, *Quantitative ultrasound of the heel and fracture risk assessment: an updated meta-analysis.* Osteoporosis Int, 2012. **23**: p. 143-53.

169.   Chan, M, Nguyen ND, Center JR, Eisman JA, Nguyen TV, *Absolute fracture-risk prediction by a combination of calcaneal quantitative ultrasound and bone mineral density.* Calcif. Tissue Int., 2012. **90**: p. 128-36.

170.   Avenell A, Gillespie WJ, Gillespie LD, O'Connell DL, *Vitamin D and vitamin D analogues for preventing fractures associated with involutional and post-menopausal osteoporosis (Review).* Cochrane Database of Systematic Reviews (3), 2005. **CD000227**.

171. Wells, G, Cranney A, Peterson J, Boucher M, Shea B, Welch V, Coyle D, Tugwell P, *Risedronate for the primary and secondary prevention of osteoporotic fractures in postmenopausal women.* Cochrane Database of Systematic Reviews (1), 2008. **CD004523**.

172. Wells, G, Cranney A, Peterson J, Boucher M, Shea B, Welch V, Coyle D, Tugwell P, *Alendronate for the primary and secondary prevention of osteoporotic fractures in postmenopausal women (review).* Cochrane Database of Systematic Reviews (1), 2008. **CD001155**.

173. National Osteoporosis Foundation, *Clinician's Guide to Prevention and Treatment of Osteoporosis,* National Osteoporosis Foundation, Editor. 2010: Washington, DC.

174. Wen, C, Wai JP, Tsai MK, et.al., *Minimum amount of physical activity for reduced mortality and extended life expectancy: a prospective cohort study.* Lancet, 2011. **378(9798)**(1244-53).

175. Sundell, J, *Resistance training is an effective tool against metabolic and frailty syndromes.* Adv Prev Med, 2011. **2011**: p. 984683.

176. Warner, S, Shea JE, Miller SC, Shaw JM, *Adaptations in cortical and trabecular bone in response to mechanical loading with and without weight bearing.* Calcif. Tissue Int., 2001. **79**(6): p. 395-403.

177. Greenway, K, Walkley JW, Rich PA, *Does long-term swimming participation have a deleterious effect on the adult female skeleton?* Eur J Appl Physiol, 2012. **Epub** (Jan 10).

178. Hans, D, Genton L, Drezner MK, Schott AM, Pacifici R, et.al., *Monitored impact loading of the hip: initial testing of a home-use device.* Calcif. Tissue Int., 2002. **71**: p. 112-20.

179. Wysocki, A, Butler M, Shamliyan T, Kane RL, *Whole-body vibration therapy for osteoporosis: state of the science.* Ann Int Med, 2011. **155**(10): p. 680-6.

180. Mikhael, M, Orr R, Singh MAF, *The effect of whole body vibration exposure on muscle or bone morphology and function in older adults: a systematic review of the literature.* Maturitas, 2010. **66**: p. 150-7.

181. Merriman, H, Jackson K, *The effects of whole-body vibration training in aging adults: a systematic review.* J. Geriatric Phys. Ther., 2009. **32**: p. 134-45.

182. Kasturi, G, Adler RA, *Osteoporosis: nonpharmacologic management* PM R, 2010. **3**(6): p. 562-72.

183. Von Stengel, S, Kemmler W, Bebenek M, Engelke K, Kalender WA, *Effects of whole-body vibration training on different devices on bone mineral density.* Med Sci Sports Exerc, 2011. **43**(6): p. 1071-9.

184. Hidalgo, JL-T, *Prevention of falls and fractures in old people by administration of calcium and vitamin D. Randomized clinical trial.* BMC Public Health, 2011. **11**: p. 910.

185. Clyburn, T, Heydemann JA, *Fall prevention in the elderly: analysis and comprehensive review of methods used in the hospital and in the home.* J Am Acad Orthop Surg, 2011. **19**: p. 402-9.

186. Gschwind, Y, Wolf I, Bridenbaugh SA, Kressig RW, *Basis for a Swiss perspective on fall prevention in vulnerable older people.* Swiss Med Wkly, 2011. **141**: p. w13305.

187. Stevens, J, Olson S, *Reducing falls and resulting hip fractures among older women,* in *MMWR (Morbidity and Mortality Weekly Report),* CDC, Editor. 2000: Washington. p. 1-12.

188. Gehrig, L, Lane J, O'Connor MI, *Osteoporosis: management and treatment strategies for orthopedic surgeons.* J. Bone Joint Surg., 2008. **90A**: p. 1362-74.

189. Farvus, M, *Bisphosphonates for osteoporosis.* NEJM, 2010. **303**(21): p. 2027-35.

190. Montori, V, Shah ND, Pencille LJ, Branda ME, Van Houten HK, Swiglo BA, et.al., *Use of a decision aid to improve treatment decisions in osteoporosis: the osteoporosis choice randomized trial.* Am J Med, 2011. **124**: p. 549-56.

191. Briesacher, B, Andrade SE, Harrod LR, Fouayzi MS, Yood RA, *Adoption of once-monthly oral bisphosphonates and the impact on adherence.* Am J Med, 2010. **123**(3): p. 275-80.

192. Gallagher, J, Levine JP, *Preventing osteoporosis in symptomatic postmenopausal women.* Menopause, 2011. **18**(1): p. 109-18.

193. Filluel, O, Crompot E, Saussez S, *Bisphosphonate-induced osteonecrosis of th jaw: a review of 2,400 patient cases.* J. Cancer Res Clin Oncol, 2010. **136**(8): p. 1117-24.

194. Bolland MJ, Grey AB, Gamble GD, Reid IR, *Effect of osteoporosis treatment on mortality: a Meta-analysis.* J Clin Endocrinol Metab, 2010. **95**: p. 1174-81.

195. Weaver, J, Miller MA, Vrahas MS, *The orthopedic implications of diphosphonate therapy.* J. Am. Acad. Orthop. Surg., 2010. **18**(6): p. 367-74.

196.   Shifren, J, Schiff I, *Role of hormone therapy in the management of menopause.* Obstet. Gynecol., 2010. **115**: p. 839-55.

197.   Saag, K, Geusens P, *Progress in osteoporosis and fracture prevention: focus on postmenopausal women.* Arth. Res. Ther., 2009. **11**: p. 251-69.

198.   Chesnut, C, Azria M, Silverman S, Engelhardt M, Olson M, Mindeholm L, *Salmon calcitonin: a review of current and future therapeutic indications.* Osteoporosis Int, 2008. **19**: p. 479-91.

199.   Cadarette, S, Katz JN, Brookhart MA, Sturmer T, Stedman MR, Solomon DH, *Relative effectiveness of osteoporosis drugs for preventing nonvertebral fractures.* Ann. Intern. Med., 2008. **148**: p. 637-46.

200.   Cummings SR, M.J., McClung MR, Siris ES, Eastell R, et.al., *Denosumab for prevention of fractures in postmenopausal women with osteoporosis.* NEJM, 2009. **361**(8): p. 756-65.

201.   Hopkins, R, Goeree R, Pullenayegum E, Adachi JD, Papaaioannou A, Xie F, Thabane L, *The relative efficacy of nine osteoporosis medications for reducing the rate of fractures in post-menopausal women.* BMC Musculoskel. Disorders, 2011. **12**: p. 209.

202.   Tosi, L, Childich R, Kannan K, Koval KJ, *The American Orthopaedic Association's "own the bone." initiative to prevent secondary fractures.* J. Bone and Joint Surg, 2008. **90**(1): p. 163-73.

203.   United States Department of Agriculture, *Dietary Guidelines for Americans, 2010. U.S. Department of Agriculture. Available at: www.dietaryguidelines.gov[Assessed February 16, 2011].* 2010: Washington.

Can You Feel It in Your Bones?